Coronary CT Angiography in the Quantitative Analysis of Coronary Plaques

Coronary CT Angiography in the Quantitative Analysis of Coronary Plaques

Zhonghua Sun
Curtin University, Australia

World Scientific

NEW JERSEY · LONDON · SINGAPORE · BEIJING · SHANGHAI · HONG KONG · TAIPEI · CHENNAI · TOKYO

Published by

World Scientific Publishing Co. Pte. Ltd.
5 Toh Tuck Link, Singapore 596224
USA office: 27 Warren Street, Suite 401-402, Hackensack, NJ 07601
UK office: 57 Shelton Street, Covent Garden, London WC2H 9HE

British Library Cataloguing-in-Publication Data
A catalogue record for this book is available from the British Library.

ISBN 978-981-4725-61-3

For any available supplementary material, please visit
http://www.worldscientific.com/worldscibooks/10.1142/9831#t=suppl

Typeset by Stallion Press
Email: enquiries@stallionpress.com

Contents

Preface

Invasive coronary angiography is the standard reference for the diagnosis of patients with suspected coronary artery disease, however, its diagnostic accuracy is being challenged by the widespread use of coronary computed tomography (CT) angiography. In addition to its invasive nature, high expense, and small procedure-related complications, invasive coronary angiography suffers from the limitation in only visualizing coronary lumen changes, while fails to provide details of plaque features or components. This has been addressed by coronary CT angiography which shows superior advantages in quantitative assessment of coronary plaques.

Coronary CT angiography has undergone rapid developments over the last decade with applications ranging from the previous focus on coronary lumen assessment to the currently functional assessment of coronary lesions, with the aim of detecting lesion-specific ischemia caused by coronary plaques. This has significant clinical impact as coronary CT angiography-derived functional analysis of coronary plaques offers insights into identification of high-risk plaques which are associated with occurrence of adverse cardiac events, and development of effective strategies for patient management. This book fulfils this goal.

This book serves as a valuable piece of literature for improving understanding of the diagnostic value of coronary CT angiography, in particular quantitative assessment of coronary plaques in relation to its clinical significance in detecting high-risk patients. Given the increasing applications of coronary CT angiography in the daily clinical practice, it is important to understand its advantages and limitations, thus achieving the goal of judicious use of coronary CT angiography in selected patients for achieving the best clinical outcomes. This is the primary intention to write this book which provides a comprehensive overview of the coronary CT angiography in the diagnostic assessment of coronary plaques, and coronary CT angiography-derived hemodynamic analysis of coronary stenosis.

The book consists of 7 chapters covering different topics related to the coronary CT angiography technical developments, recent dose-reduction strategies, image processing and visualization of coronary plaques and coronary CT angiography-derived hemodynamics. Chapter 1 is an introduction of the increasing applications of coronary CT angiography in the diagnosis of coronary artery disease and a brief outline of each chapter. Chapter 2 describes the commonly used scanning techniques of coronary CT angiography with a focus on dose-reduction strategies. Latest technical developments such as iterative reconstruction and automatic motion correction algorithms are covered as well. Chapter 3 discusses the 2D and 3D visualizations of coronary plaques, with inclusion of quantitative assessment of coronary plaques by comparing coronary CT angiography with intravascular ultrasound. Automatic quantification of coronary plaques is also discussed in this chapter. Chapter 4 emphasizes the quantitative assessment of coronary plaque features by coronary CT angiography with the aim of quantifying these plaque characteristics in terms of vulnerability and association with major cardiac events. Chapters 5 and 6 focus on coronary CT angiography-derived flow dynamic analysis. Chapter 5 mainly presents an overview of coronary CT angiography-generated 3D models for hemodynamic analysis, while Chapter 6 provides a comprehensive review of the coronary CT angiography-derived fractional flow reserve which is currently a hot topic, with evidence supported by the current literature. Chapter 7 is a brief summary and conclusions of the diagnostic performance of coronary CT angiography in coronary artery disease.

The main driving force of CT developments is owing to the wide availability of CT scanners and extensive use of cardiac CT imaging, which requires superior spatial and temporal resolution for accurate diagnosis of coronary artery disease. Technological advancements in coronary CT angiography have enabled this technique to not only demonstrate excellent coronary anatomy with high precision, but also provide functional assessment of coronary stenosis with the ability of detecting lesion-specific ischemia. Quantitative assessment of coronary plaques by coronary CT angiography along with computational fluid dynamics allows detection of vulnerable plaques, thus developing personalized medicine to treat individual patients with effective outcomes.

This book is intended primarily for cardiologists, radiologists, medical imaging scientists and postgraduate research students who show strong research and clinical interests in coronary CT angiography and coronary plaque imaging. It is expected that this book will further enhance understanding of the diagnostic performance of coronary CT angiography in the quantitative assessment of coronary plaques and maximize the clinical impact of coronary CT angiography.

Zhonghua Sun, MB, PhD, FSCCT, FRSM

1 Introduction

Coronary artery disease (CAD) is the leading cause of morbidity and mortality in developed countries and its prevalence is increasing in developing countries. Invasive coronary angiography (ICA) is the gold standard for accurate assessment of coronary anatomy changes and diagnosis of CAD due to its superior spatial and temporal resolution which allows for accurate identification and assessment of degree of lumen stenosis resulting from obstructive coronary lesions. However, a major limitation of ICA is that it is a "luminogram", thus, providing little information about plaque morphological features/plaque components or coronary wall changes, both of which play an important role in determining plaque vulnerability.[1] This results in low sensitivity and specificity for the early detection of the vulnerable plaque by ICA.

The most important role of radiological imaging in the diagnostic assessment of CAD is to analyze imaging features of CAD with the aim of determining the risk of plaque rupture since there is a poor correlation between coronary lumen stenosis and functional/hemodynamic significance. In addition to the routine diagnosis of the degree of lumen stenosis,[2-5] quantitative assessment of the morphological characteristics including presence of calcification within plaque,[6-9] complex lesions with plaque disruption and thrombosis,[10,11] and coronary artery movement patterns has become part of coronary plaque imaging evaluation.[12,13]

ICA is unable to provide information about the morphology or plaque composition such as non-calcified plaque, or large lipid-rich core indicating vulnerable plaque, or other histological characteristics including thin fibrous cap, plaque erosion, and neoangiogenesis.[14,15] Current evidence

1

Table 1.1. Advantages and limitations of ICA in coronary plaque assessment (modified from Chan and Ng[1]).

Plaque characteristics	Ability to detect or diagnose (references)
Degree of stenosis	Yes with high precision[2–4]
Vessel wall	No
Plaque composition	No
Plaque volume	No
Fibrous cap or lipid core thickness	No
Thrombus within plaque	Possibly[10,11]
Calcium within plaque	Possibly[6–9]
Ruptured plaque	Possibly[10,11]
Coronary artery movement	Yes[2,12,13]

shows that although ICA is the standard reference for diagnostic assessment of coronary lumen irregularities, it has limited value for determining coronary plaque features.[1,10] Table 1.1 summarizes the advantages and limitations of ICA in the diagnosis of various plaque features.

The established role of ICA in the diagnosis of CAD is gradually losing when compared to other imaging modalities such as coronary computed tomography angiography (CCTA) or intravascular ultrasound which is able to look beyond the coronary lumen changes, thus allowing for both anatomic detection and hemodynamic evaluation of CAD.[16] Rapid technological advancements in CT scanners have enabled the widespread use of CCTA for the non-invasive assessment of CAD with high accuracy because of excellent quality images, even in patients with high heart rates. CT scanners that are post-64 and have more detector rows are available worldwide, with studies reporting the superior diagnostic value of CCTA in the detection of significant CAD with ICA as the reference method.[17–23] In particular, the very high negative predictive value of CCTA (>95%) indicates that it can be used as a reliable imaging modality for exclusion of significant CAD, thus, avoiding unnecessary downstream imaging tests or invasive procedures in patients with low to intermediate risk of CAD.

CCTA allows evaluation of coronary plaque imaging features.[24,25] Classification of coronary plaque compositions by CCTA has demonstrated important clinical implications, because there is significant association of plaque components with myocardial ischemia and prevalence of adverse major cardiac events and prediction of CAD prognosis.[26–29] The recently introduced semi-quantitative and automatic quantitative plaques assessment tools further advance the diagnostic value of CCTA through characterizing and quantifying coronary plaques with high intra- and inter-observer reproducibility.[30,31] There is a growing body of evidence showing that CCTA has incremental prognostic value over traditional risk factors.[32,33] Furthermore, CCTA combined with computational fluid dynamics, or CCTA-derived fractional flow reserve (FFR_{CT}) has further advanced the diagnostic performance of CCTA to determine the physiological significance of coronary stenosis, therefore, improving clinical decision-making and clinical outcome through identification of coronary lesions that result in myocardial ischemia.[34–38] Analysis of coronary lesions by CCTA providing both anatomic and functional information represents the current research direction in quantitative assessment of coronary plaques, and this is the main focus of this book.

The following chapters will provide a comprehensive overview of CCTA with regard to its clinical applications in the quantitative assessment of coronary plaques. Chapter 2 focuses on technical developments in CCTA including recently introduced various dose-saving strategies, while Chapter 3 provides an overview of 2D and 3D characterization of coronary plaques by CCTA with a focus on quantitative assessment of plaque features with the aim of identifying vulnerable plaques. Chapter 4 focuses on CCTA quantitative analysis of various plaques. Chapters 5 and 6 discuss the functional assessment of coronary plaques including CCTA-derived computational fluid dynamics and FFR_{CT}. Chapter 6 provides an updated overview of the current evidence of FFR_{CT} in the detection of coronary plaques, especially lesion-specific ischemia based on multicenter, single-center studies as well as systematic reviews and meta-analyses. Chapter 7 is a summary and conclusion of the clinical value of CCTA in CAD.

References

1. Chan KH, Ng MKC. (2013) Is there a role for coronary angiography in the early detection of vulnerable plaque? *Int J Cardiol* **164**: 262–266.
2. Chan K, Chawantanpipat C, Gattorna T *et al.* (2010) The relationship between coronary stenosis severity and compression type coronary artery movement in acute myocardial infarction. *Am Heart J* **159**: 584–592.

3. Frøbert O, van't Veer M, Aarnoudse W, Simonsen U, Koolen J, Pijls N. (2007) Acute myocardial infarction and underlying stenosis severity. *Catheter Cardiovasc Interv* **70**: 958–965.

4. Manoharan G, Ntalianis A, Muller O *et al.* (2009) Severity of coronary arterial stenoses responsible for acute coronary syndromes. *Am J Cardiol* **103**: 1183–1188.

5. Little W, Constantinescu M, Applegate R *et al.* (1988) Can coronary angiography predict the site of a subsequent myocardial infarction in patients with mild-to-moderate coronary artery disease? *Circulation* **78**: 1157–1166.

6. Burke A, Taylor A, Farb A, Malcom G, Virmani R. (2000) Coronary calcification: insights from sudden coronary death victims. *Z Kardiol* **89**: 49–53.

7. Cheng G, Loree H, Kamm R, Fishbein M, Lee R. (1993) Distribution of circumferential stress in ruptured and stable atherosclerotic lesions: a structural analysis with histopathological correlation. *Circulation* **87**: 1179–1187.

8. Margolis J, Chen J, Kong Y, Peter R, Behar V, Kisslo J. (1980) The diagnostic and prognostic significance of coronary artery calcification. A report of 800 cases. *Radiology* **137**: 609.

9. Rasheed Q, Nair R, Sheehan H, Hodgson J. (1994) Correlation of intracoronary ultrasound plaque characteristics in atherosclerotic coronary artery disease patients with clinical variables. *Am J Cardiol* **73**: 753–758.

10. Levin D, Fallon J. (1982) Significance of the angiographic morphology of localized coronary stenoses: histopathologic correlations. *Circulation* **66**: 316–320.

11. Waxman S, Mittleman M, Zarich S *et al.* (2003) Plaque disruption and thrombus in Ambrose's angiographic coronary lesion types. *Am J Cardiol* **92**: 16–20.

12. Konta T, Bett J. (2003) Patterns of coronary artery movement and the development of coronary atherosclerosis. *Circ J* **67**: 846–850.

13. O'Loughlin A, Byth K. (2007) The stretch-compression type of coronary artery movement predicts the location of culprit lesions responsible for ST-segment elevation myocardial infarctions. *Heart Lung Circ* **16**: 265–268.

14. Naghavi M, Libby P, Falk E *et al.* (2003) From vulnerable plaque to vulnerable patient — a call for new definitions and risk assessment strategies: part I. *Circulation* **108**: 1664–1672.

15. Virmani R, Kolodgie F, Burke A, Farb A, Schwartz S. (2000) Lessons from sudden coronary death — a comprehensive morphological classification scheme for atherosclerotic lesions. *Arterioscler Thromb Vasc Biol* **20**: 1262–1275.

16. Colombo A, Panoulas VF. (2015) Diagnostic coronary angiography is getting old! *JACC Cardiovasc Imaging* **8**: 11–13.

17. Budoff MJ, Achenbach S, Blumenthal RS *et al.* (2006) Assessment of coronary artery disease by cardiac computed tomography: a scientific statement from the American Heart Association Committee on Cardiovascular Imaging and Intervention, Council on Cardiovascular Radiology and Intervention, and Committee on Cardiac Imaging, Council on Clinical Cardiology. *Circulation* **114**(16): 1761–1791.

18. Miller JM, Rochitte CE, Dewey M *et al.* (2008) Diagnostic performance of coronary angiography by 64-row CT. *N Engl J Med* **359**(22): 2324–2336.

19. Budoff MJ, Dowe D, Jollis JG *et al.* (2008) Diagnostic performance of 64-multidetector row coronary computed tomographic angiography for evaluation of coronary artery stenosis in individuals without known coronary artery disease: results from the prospective multicenter ACCURACY (Assessment by Coronary Computed Tomographic Angiography of Individuals Undergoing Invasive Coronary Angiography) trial. *J Am Coll Cardiol* **52**(21): 1724–1732.

20. Schroeder S, Achenbach S, Bengel F *et al.* (2008) Cardiac computed tomography: indications, applications, limitations, and training requirements — report of a writing group deployed by the Working Group Nuclear Cardiology and Cardiac CT of the European Society of Cardiology and the European Council of Nuclear Cardiology. *Eur Heart J* **29**(4): 531–556.

21. Sun Z, Lin C. (2014) Diagnostic value of 320-slice coronary CT angiography in coronary artery disease: a systematic review and meta-analysis. *Curr Med Imaging Rev* **10**: 272–280.

22. Sun Z, Almoudi M, Cao Y. (2014) CT angiography in the diagnosis of cardiovascular disease: a transformation in cardiovascular CT practice. *Quant Imaging Med Surg* **4**: 376–396.

23. Machida H, Tanaka I, Fukui R *et al.* (2015) Current and novel imaging techniques in coronary CT. *Radiographics* **356**: 991–1010.

24. Foster G, Shah H, Sarraf G, Ahmadi N, Budoff M. (2009) Detection of noncalcified and mixed plaque by multirow detector computed tomography. *Expert Rev Cardiovasc Ther* **7**: 57–64.

25. Sun Z, Xu L. (2014) Coronary CT angiography in the quantitative assessment of coronary plaques. *Biomed Res Int* **2014**: 346380.

26. Pundziute G, Schuijf JD, Jukema JW *et al.* (2008) Head-to-head comparison of coronary plaque evaluation between multislice computed tomography and intravascular ultrasound radiofrequency data analysis. *JACC Cardiovasc Interv* **1**: 76–82.

27. Lin F, Shaw LJ, Berman DS *et al.* (2008) Multidetector computed tomography coronary artery plaque predictors of stress-induced myocardial ischemia by SPECT. *Atherosclerosis* **197**: 700–709.

28. Pundziute G, Schuijf JD, Jukema JW *et al.* (2007) Prognostic value of multislice computed tomography coronary angiography in patients with known or suspected coronary artery disease. *J Am Coll Cardiol* **49**: 62–70.

29. van Werkhoven JM, Schuijf JD, Gaemperli O *et al.* (2009) Prognostic value of multislice computed tomography and gated single-photon emission computed tomography in patients with suspected coronary artery disease. *J Am Coll Cardiol* **53**: 623–632.

30. Rinehart S, Vazquez G, Qian Z, Murrieta L, Christian K, Voros S. (2011) Quantitative measurements of coronary arterial stenosis, plaque geometry, and composition are highly reproducible with a standardized coronary arterial computed tomographic approach in high-quality CT datasets. *J Cardiovasc Comput Tomogr* **5**: 35–43.

31. Diaz-Zamudio M, Dey D, Schuhbaeck A *et al.* (2015) Automated quantitative plaque burden from coronary CT angiography noninvasively predicts hemodynamic significance by using fractional flow reserve in intermediate coronary lesions. *Radiology* **276**: 408–415.

32. Sun Z, Wang YL, Hsieh IC, Liu YC, Wen MS. (2013) Coronary CT angiography in the diagnosis of coronary artery disease. *Curr Med Imaging Rev* **9**: 184–193.

33. Miszalski-Jamka T, Klimeczek P, Banys R *et al.* (2012) The composition and extent of coronary artery plaque detected by multislice computed tomographic angiography provides incremental prognostic value in patients with suspected coronary artery disease. *Int J Cardiovasc Imaging* **28**: 621–631.

34. Xu L, Sun Z, Fan Z. (2014) Noninvasive physiologic assessment of coronary stenoses using cardiac CT. *Biomed Res Int* **2014**: 435737.

35. George RT, Mehra VC, Chen MY *et al.* (2014) Myocardial CT perfusion imaging and SPECT for the diagnosis of coronary artery disease: a head-to-head comparison from the CORE320 multicenter diagnostic performance study. *Radiology* **272**: 407–416.

36. Keirns CC, Goold SD. (2009) Patient-centered care and preference-sensitive decision making. *JAMA* **302**: 1805–1806.

37. Sun Z. (2015) Evidence for myocardial CT perfusion imaging in the diagnosis of hemodynamically significant coronary artery disease. *Cardiovasc Diag Ther* **5**: 58–62.

38. Sun Z, Xu L. (2014) Computational fluid dynamics in coronary artery diseases. *Comput Med Imaging Graph* **38**: 651–663.

2 Coronary CT Angiography: Technological Developments

Table of Contents

Abstract

Coronary CT angiography (CCTA) is a widely used less-invasive imaging modality for diagnostic assessment of coronary artery disease with high diagnostic value. Technical developments have rapidly evolved in recent years to overcome limitations of conventional CCTA, in particular further lowering radiation dose and improving diagnostic performance. This chapter focuses on the recent and novel imaging techniques that are used in CCTA. It is clinically important to understand these techniques for enhancing the diagnostic performance of CCTA while minimizing radiation exposure to patients.

Keywords: coronary CT angiography, image quality, radiation dose, spatial resolution, temporal resolution, technological developments.

2.1 Introduction

Since the advent of multislice CT nearly two decades ago, continuous and significant improvements have taken place in the technical capabilities of this fast evolving technique. The progress of multislice CT is demonstrated by the increasing role of non-invasive coronary CT angiography (CCTA) in the detection and diagnosis of coronary artery disease (CAD) and the high accuracy achieved with the current multislice CT scanners.[1–6]

Technical advancements of multislice CT from the early generation of 4-slice scanners to the current 320- and 640-slice scanners have significantly improved the spatial resolution, which allows for acquisition of isotropic data ($0.35 \times 0.35 \times 0.35$ mm^3) for accurate assessment of coronary anatomical details including plaque assessment.[7,8] High temporal resolution is another critical factor for "freezing" the movement of coronary arteries during cardiac cycle, thus enabling the capture of cardiac images without their being affected by motion-related artifacts. The temporal resolution has been significantly increased from the 250 ms in 4-slice CT scanners to 165 ms in 64-slice scanners and 66 ms in dual-source CT (DSCT) scanners.[9–13] Although still inferior to that of invasive coronary angiography (ICA) (10–20 ms), the improved temporal resolution in multislice CT scanners with similar spatial resolution to that of ICA (0.23 mm vs 0.2 mm) enables acquisition of high-quality images, even in patients with high heart rates.

Despite these promising results, CCTA examinations expose patients to a nephrotoxic contrast medium that could induce renal damage, leading to renal dysfunction, which is commonly referred to as contrast-induced nephropathy (CIN) or acute kidney injury. Another limitation of CCTA lies in the radiation exposure, which is associated with carcinogenic development. A number of strategies or imaging techniques have been developed to address these limitations during CCTA examinations, with satisfactory results having been achieved. These technological developments include the use of prospective electrocardiography (ECG)-triggered and high-pitch CCTA to lower radiation dose to the submillisievert level; application of automatic tube potential and iterative reconstruction (IR) for further reducing dose without compromising image quality; high-definition CT to improve spatial resolution and dual-energy CT (DECT) for acquisition of both anatomic and functional information; and automatic correction algorithms for minimizing cardiac motion-related artifacts.[9–23] This chapter provides an overview of these technical developments that are currently used in CCTA.

2.2 Prospective ECG Triggering (Axial and Helical Scans)

Cardiac CT imaging is different from non-cardiac CT scans since monitoring the cardiac cycle with ECG recording during scanning allows acquisition of synchronized images and reconstruction of images at the optimal cardiac phase to minimize motion artifacts arising from high or irregular heartbeats. The standard, retrospectively ECG-gated helical CCTA is performed with a highly overlapping scan with a very low pitch (0.2–0.4) to ensure coverage of the entire heart, thus enabling acquisition of volumetric data for selection of the reconstruction window throughout the cardiac phase. However, this technique suffers from high radiation dose due to the same anatomic area being exposed to X-ray radiation during consecutive rotations of the gantry with use of low pitch value. Furthermore, in many patients, especially those with a low or regular heart rate, it is unnecessary to acquire other phases because reconstruction of CCTA imaging data can be achieved during the diastolic phase. This leads to the increasing use of prospectively ECG-triggered approach.

The principle of prospective ECG triggering is that data acquisition only takes place at a predetermined cardiac phase (most commonly during diastolic phase) by selectively turning on the X-ray beam when triggered by the ECG signal to acquire sufficient data for reconstruction of images during the minimal acquisition window, and turning off the X-ray beam during systolic phase. This technical approach is different from the retrospectively ECG-gated helical CCTA because it significantly reduces radiation dose by limiting the number of cardiac phases for data acquisition and by increasing the pitch to 1.0, with no overlapping with the following scan.[14,24] Although prospective ECG triggering does not provide functional myocardial information, which is one of the main limitations of this protocol, this has been addressed by the emergence of newer CT scanners such as 256- and 320-slice CT that allow for extended longitudinal coverage of the anatomic region.

Many studies have confirmed the effectiveness of dose reduction with use of prospectively ECG-triggered CCTA, while in the meantime acquiring high diagnostic value for detection of CAD.[10–13] The effective radiation dose is reported to range from 2 to 6 mSv with the prospective ECG triggering, and it has similar or improved image quality compared with that of the retrospectively ECG-gated protocol (Fig. 2.1) (Table 2.1).[25–31] According to several systematic reviews and meta-analyses, CCTA performed with prospective ECG triggering has high diagnostic performance

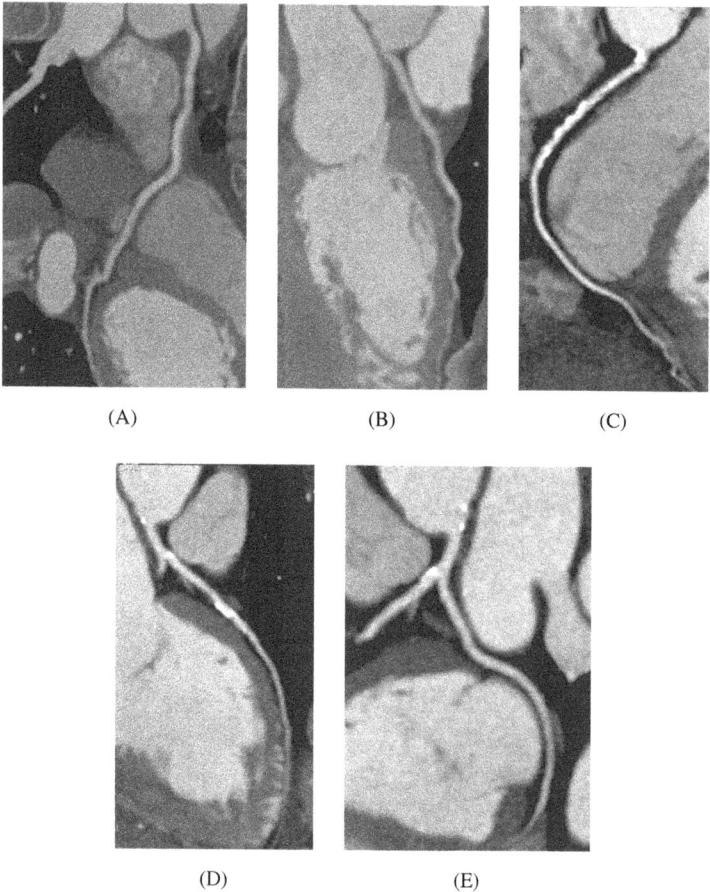

(A)   (B)   (C)

(D)   (E)

Figure 2.1. Prospectively ECG-triggered CCTA shows normal right coronary artery (A) and left anterior descending artery (B). In another patient, prospectively ECG-triggered CCTA shows multiple calcified plaques at the right coronary artery (C), left anterior descending (D) and left circumflex (E) with excellent visualization of both normal anatomy and atherosclerotic changes.

Table 2.1. Prospectively ECG-triggered CCTA in coronary artery disease according to systematic reviews and meta-analyses.

First author	No. of articles in the analysis	Pooled sensitivity (95% CI)			Pooled specificity (95% CI)			Radiation dose (mSv) (95% CI)
		Patient-based	Vessel-based	Segment-based	Patient-based	Vessel-based	Segment-based	
Von Ballmoos et al.[10]	16 studies	100% (98–100)	97% (95–98)	91% (86–95)	89% (82–89)	93% (89–96)	96% (94–97)	2.7 (2.2, 3.2)
Sun et al.[11]	14 studies	99% (98–100)	95% (93–96)	92% (90–93)	91% (88–94)	95% (93–95)	97% (97–98)	3.3 (2.3, 4.1)
Sun et al.[12]	22 studies	97.7% (93.7–100)	N/A	N/A	92.1% (87.2–97)	N/A	N/A	4.5 (3.6, 5.3)
Sabarudin et al.[13]	23 studies	98.3% (96–100)	89.3% (79.6–99)	89.8% (76.6–98)	90.5% (85.7–96)	94.7% (92.3–97)	97.2% (95–98.5)	3.6 (2.9, 4.3)
Yang et al.[32]	12 studies	100% (98–100)	98% (96–99)	93% (88–97)	89% (85–92)	93% (88–96)	96% (94–98)	2.1 (1.7, 3.1)
Menke et al.[33]	20 studies	98.7% (95.5–99.6)	N/A	91.3% (82.4–96)	91.3% (81.7–96.1)	N/A	97.7% (96.6–98.5)	3.5 (3.0, 4.1)

Note: N/A: not available.

with mean sensitivity and specificity ranging from 99% to 100% and 89% to 91% on per-patient-based analysis, and 95% to 97% and 93% to 95%; 91% to 92% and 96% to 97%, on per-vessel and per-segment-based analysis, respectively.[10–13,32,33] Further dose reduction can be achieved with lower kVp values, such as 100 or 80, or even 70 kVp.[34,35] Therefore, a combination of prospective ECG triggering with a low kVp protocol is currently recommended in patients with body mass index (BMI) less than 25 kg/m^2, since changing tube voltage needs to be correlated with the patient's BMI. This will be further discussed in the following sections.

Prospective ECG triggering is mainly limited to patients with low and regular heart rates (heart rates less than 70 beats per minute (bpm)) or low heart rate variability and without arrhythmias. In patients with higher or irregular heart rates, use of prospective ECG triggering is also feasible, but at the expense of higher radiation dose due to the use of padding.[36–38] The developments of DSCT scanners enable prospectively ECG-triggered CCTA to be performed with high-pitch helical protocol, achieving very low dose.[39–43] The second generation of DSCT scanners (Siemens Definition Flash) with acquisition of 128 slices per rotation, and the third generation of DSCT scanners (Siemens Somatom Force) with acquisition of 192 slices per rotation have made high-pitch protocols (pitch value up to 3.4) possible, with radiation dose further being lowered to less than 1 mSv. In their recent study, Goric et al. showed that prospectively ECG-triggered CCTA with use of the third-generation DSCT with high-pitch mode produced high diagnostic image quality in patients with heart rates less than 70 bpm, but image quality of CCTA is not affected by heart rate variability.[43] The combination of this scanning protocol with lower kVp and other image post-processing algorithms has been reported to further reduce radiation dose to even less than 0.1 mSv.[44]

2.3 Automatic Tube Potential Modulation

Tremendous dose reductions have been achieved in CCTA with use of various dose-saving strategies including tube current modulation, prospective ECG-triggering and high-pitch protocols. The relationship between tube potential, radiation dose and image quality is more complex, with most of the previous studies adjusting tube potential based on

BMI.[45–49] According to Society of Cardiovascular Computed Tomography (SCCT) guidelines on radiation dose and dose-optimization strategies in cardiovascular CT, a tube voltage of 100 kVp is recommended for patients weighing ≤90 kg or with a BMI ≤30 kg/m^2; a tube voltage of 120 kVp is usually indicated for patients weighing >90 kg and with a BMI >30 kg/m^2. Reduction of the tube voltage to 80 kVp should only be considered in children and slim young adults with BMI below 20 kg/m^2.[50] The updated SCCT guidelines revised these recommendations with the following suggestions: 80 kVp is recommended in patients with BMI <18 kg/m^2; 100 kVp is recommended in patients with BMI <30 kg/m^2; 120 kVp is recommended in patients with BMI between 30 and 40 kg/m^2 and 140 kVp is recommended in patients with BMI >40 kg/m^2. [51]

However, chest size is not always concordant with BMI or body weight as there is a high rate of disagreement between BMI and chest size. Ghoshhajra et al. reported 39% discordance between BMI and chest size in their study after analyzing 182 patients who underwent CCTA.[52] Using BMI to select tube potential could lead to overdosing or underdosing during CCTA; thus, the authors suggested that using chest area to choose tube potential might serve as a more appropriate dose parameter. Recently developed automated software algorithm has been shown to improve image quality while further reducing radiation dose.

Ghoshhajra et al. in another report presented their first experience of CCTA with automatic tube potential selection in 38 patients with suspected CAD in comparison with 38 matched patients as control group who underwent CCTA with BMI used to adjust tube potential.[53] A range of kVp values from 80 to 140 were used in both groups, and subjective and objective image quality were assessed. They found significant improvements in objective image quality in the group using automatic tube selection when compared to the standard BMI-based tube selection, with 30% dose reduction in the study group compared to the control group. This has been confirmed by a recent study showing similar findings.[54] Layritz and colleagues evaluated the automated attenuation-based selection of tube voltage for CCTA in 50 patients and compared the image quality and radiation dose to the control group with 50 patients but using BMI as the criterion to select tube voltage. A dose reduction of 39% (1.4 vs 2.3 mSv) was achieved in the automatic tube selection group while still

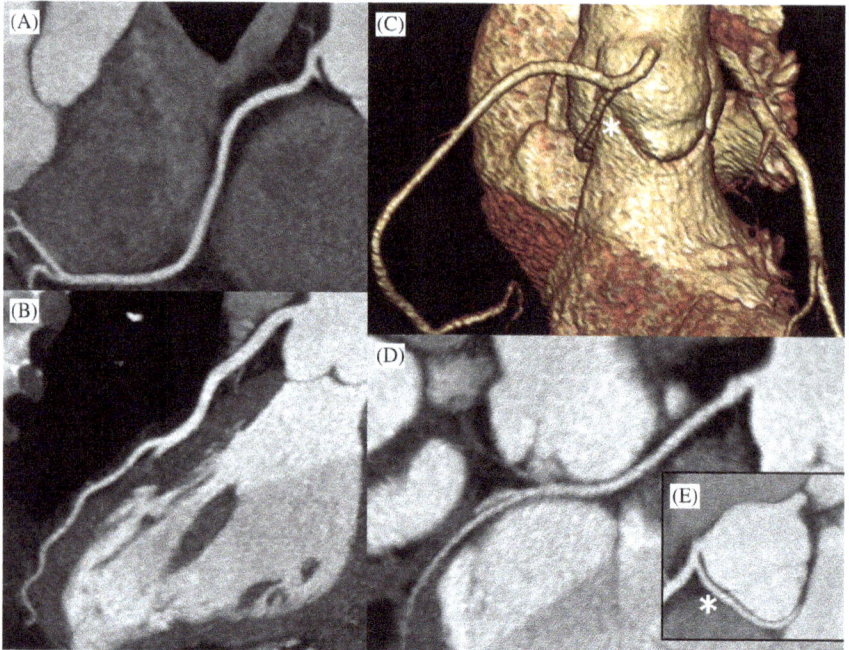

Figure 2.2. Attention-based selection of tube potential and tube current in a 45-year-old female with atypical chest pain. Tube voltage and tube current were 100 kV and 151 mAs, respectively, with resultant effective dose of 1.0 mSv. Curved planar reformatted images show three main coronary arteries without any sign of CAD (A, B, D). The left circumflex coronary artery demonstrates an anomalous course arising from the proximal right coronary artery with subsequent retro-aortic course (*) as shown in the images (C and E). Reprinted with permission from Layritz et al.[54]

maintaining diagnostic image quality (Fig. 2.2).[54] These single center-based studies show promising results of using automated tube potential selection, although further research with inclusion of a large number of patients is required.

2.4 Iterative Reconstruction (IR)

Image reconstruction algorithms play an essential role in defining the quality and integrity of cardiac CT images. CT images have been reconstructed from raw data using filtered back projection (FBP) since the introduction of CT into clinical practice. Although FBP is a fast and highly efficient algorithm in image reconstruction, it suffers from increased image noise and less image reliability.

IR is a type of reconstruction algorithm that creates cross-sectional images from measured projections of an object. IR has been used widely in emission tomographic imaging modalities such as single-photon emission computed tomography (SPECT) and positron emission tomography (PET). This algorithm was not commonly used in CT imaging mainly due to significantly slower computational speed, which limits the widespread use of this algorithm in clinical CT scanners. In recent years, the four major CT vendors have developed simplified versions of IR in cardiac CT imaging, with promising results having been reported in the literature. The currently available IR algorithms in CCTA include adaptive statistical IR (ASIR, GE Healthcare), IR in image space (IRIS, Siemens Healthcare), sonogram-affirmed IR (SAFIRE, Siemens Healthcare), IR technique (iDose, Philips Healthcare) and adaptive iterative dose reduction (AIDR, AIDR 3D, Toshiba Medical Systems),[14] while some recent advancements such as model-based IR (MBIR) or knowledge-based IR demonstrate further noise reduction and improvement in image quality with submillisievert dose.[55–57]

The major advantage of these IR algorithms lies in the reduction of radiation dose through lowering tube current without increasing image noise. Studies have shown the effectiveness in CCTA using IR for reduction of radiation dose compared to the conventional FBP-reconstructed CCTA.[58–60] Based on these single and multicenter studies, the use of IR in CCTA is shown to reduce radiation dose by up to 44% compared to the use of FBP. When IR is combined with other dose-saving strategies, such as prospective ECG-triggering, high-pitch protocol and low kVp, very low dose or even ultra-low dose CCTA can be achieved. Chen and colleagues reported their experience of using the second-generation 320-slice CT combined with IR and automatic exposure control in 107 patients with different body sizes and variable heart rates.[61] Excellent image quality was found with the median radiation dose of 0.93 mSv, which is more than a 75% reduction compared to the first-generation 320-slice CT. Further dose reduction is also possible with the use of even lower kVp. Another recent study evaluated the feasibility of lowering tube potential to 70 kVp with the third-generation DSCT.[62] Prospectively ECG-triggered

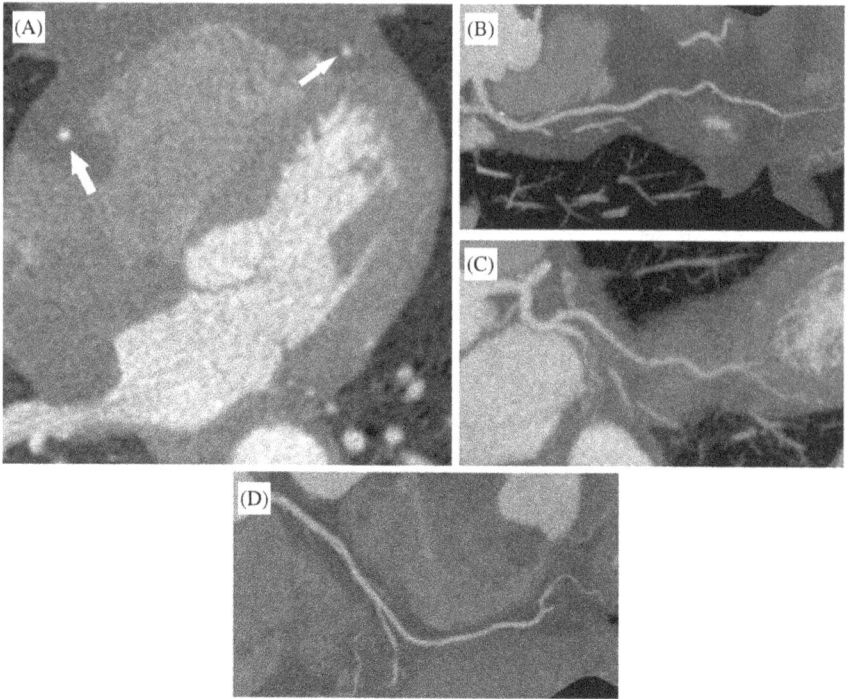

Figure 2.3. Prospectively ECG-triggered high-pitch CCTA in a 66-year-old female using a third-generation DSCT with 70 kVp and 450 mAs. A: transverse axial images at the mid-segment of right coronary artery (large arrow) and left anterior descending coronary artery (small arrow). B–D: curved planar reformations show the left anterior descending, left circumflex and right coronary artery. Images were reconstructed using FBP with slice thickness of 0.6 mm and an increment of 0.3 mm. Reprinted with permission from Hell *et al.*[62]

CCTA with high-pitch protocol was used in 26 patients with body weight <100 kg and heart rate <60 bpm, with images reconstructed using IR and FBP algorithms (Fig. 2.3). The mean radiation dose was 0.3 mSv, with better image quality and lower rate of non-diagnostic images noted in CCTA using IR compared with those using FBP (Fig. 2.4). These findings were confirmed by Meyer *et al.* who reported similar findings.[63] Third-generation DSCT at 70 kVp resulted in improved image quality and significantly lower radiation dose (0.44 vs 0.92 mSv) and contrast medium requirement (45 vs 80 mL) as compared with second-generation DSCT.

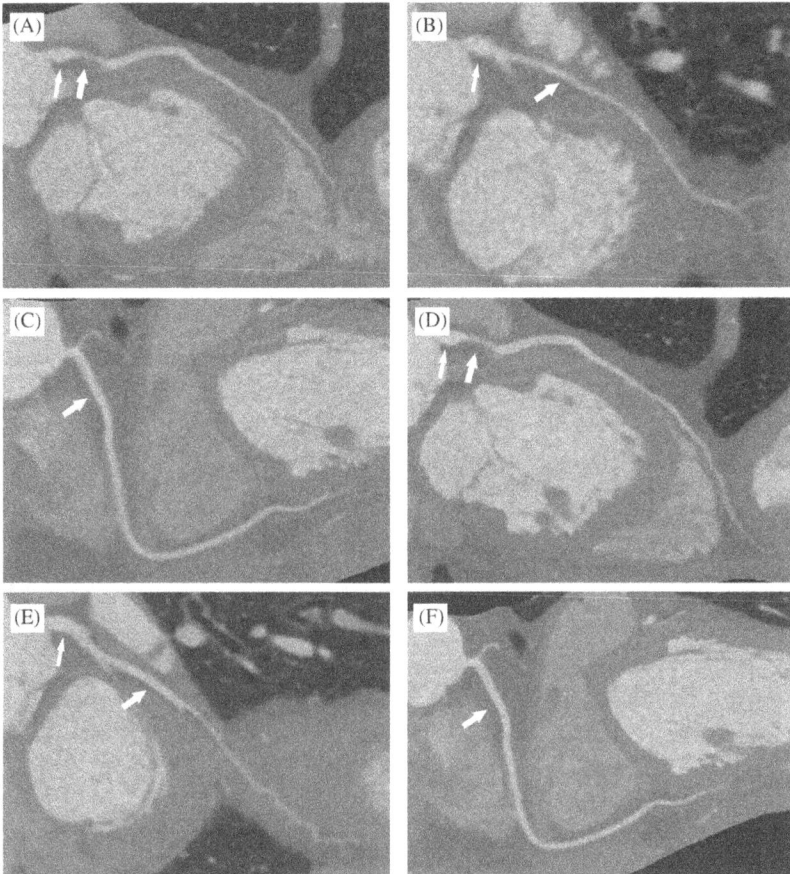

Figure 2.4. Prospectively ECG-triggered high-pitch CCTA in a 62-year-old male with 70 kVp and 450 mAs. A–C: images were reconstructed using FBP; D–F: images were reconstructed using iterative reconstruction algorithm (ADMIRE at a strength level of 2) with slice thickness of 0.6 mm and an increment of 0.3 mm. Curved planar reformatted images show high-grade stenosis at the left anterior descending (large arrow in A and D), and normal left main and left circumflex (large arrow in B and E) and right coronary arteries (small arrow in C and F). ICA confirms these findings as observed on CCTA (G–I) (large arrows point to left anterior descending, left circumflex and right coronary arteries). J: 3D volume rendering of left coronary artery with arrow indicating the high-degree stenosis in the left anterior descending coronary artery. Reprinted with permission from Hell *et al.*[62]

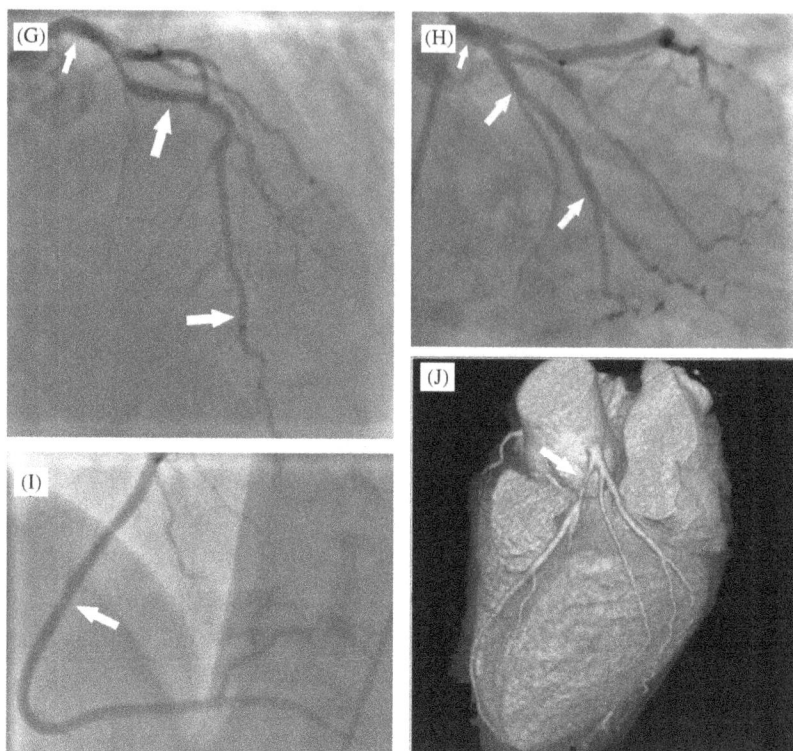

Figure 2.4. (*Continued*)

Of these raw data-based IR algorithms for noise reduction, MBIR represents a recently developed algorithm which has been shown to further reduce radiation dose.[55–57] Stehli *et al.* reported high diagnostic accuracy of CCTA using MBIR with 96.9% coronary segments being interpretable, resulting in a mean radiation dose of 0.29 mSv, which is comparable with a chest X-ray in two views.[64] Ultra-low dose CCTA is also reported in a recent study indicating that effective dose can be further reduced to less than 0.1 mSv. Schuhbaeck *et al.* used prospectively ECG-triggered high-pitch helical CCTA in 21 patients with body weight <100 kg and heart rate <60 bpm, with images reconstructed using FBP and IR.[65] The mean effective dose was 0.06 mSv in this study, with significantly lower image noise in IR. In patients with a body weight <75 kg, no significant difference was found in image quality assessment between IR- and FBP-reconstructed

CCTA images. A recent systematic review and meta-analysis has shown significant dose reduction in CCTA with use of IR compared to FBP (pooled effective dose 2.2 mSv vs 4.2 mSv for IR and FBP).[66] These early findings need to be confirmed by larger studies with a focus on evaluating diagnostic value in CAD.

Although ECG-based tube current modulation was widely used for dose reduction during CCTA examinations during early stages of cardiac CT imaging,[67] adjustment of tube current should be performed with caution due to close association between tube current and image quality. With widespread application of IR algorithms in clinical practice with significant dose reduction, tube current modulation is becoming more commonly used in combination with IR to reduce dose values, despite the presence of high heart rates.[68]

2.5 High-definition CT

High-definition or high-resolution CT is a recently introduced CT scanner (Discovery CT 750 HD, GE Healthcare) with gemstone detectors and significant improvements in the data acquisition system. High-definition CT is capable of improving spatial resolution to 0.23 mm and contrast resolution to 3 mm, which is much better than the corresponding spatial and contrast resolution of 0.33–0.50 mm and 5 mm obtained with standard CCTA.[69–71] High-definition CT has been shown to improve the diagnostic accuracy of CCTA for the assessment of significant coronary stenosis and coronary stents by minimizing the effect of blooming artifacts.

Kazakauskaite *et al.* presented the first experience of comparing high-definition CT with standard 64-slice CCTA in two groups of patients (with 93 in each group) with matched heart rate, heart rate variability and BMI.[71] Results showed no significant difference in mean image quality between the two types of CT scanners. A reduction of effective dose was found in the high-definition CT group with use of ASIR when compared to the group undergoing standard 64-slice CCTA (1.7 vs 1.9 mSv), although no diagnostic value was investigated in this study (Fig. 2.5). It is well known that the diagnostic accuracy of CCTA is limited for the assessment of calcified coronary plaques due to blooming or beam hardening artifacts resulting from the high calcium scores in the coronary artery, thus

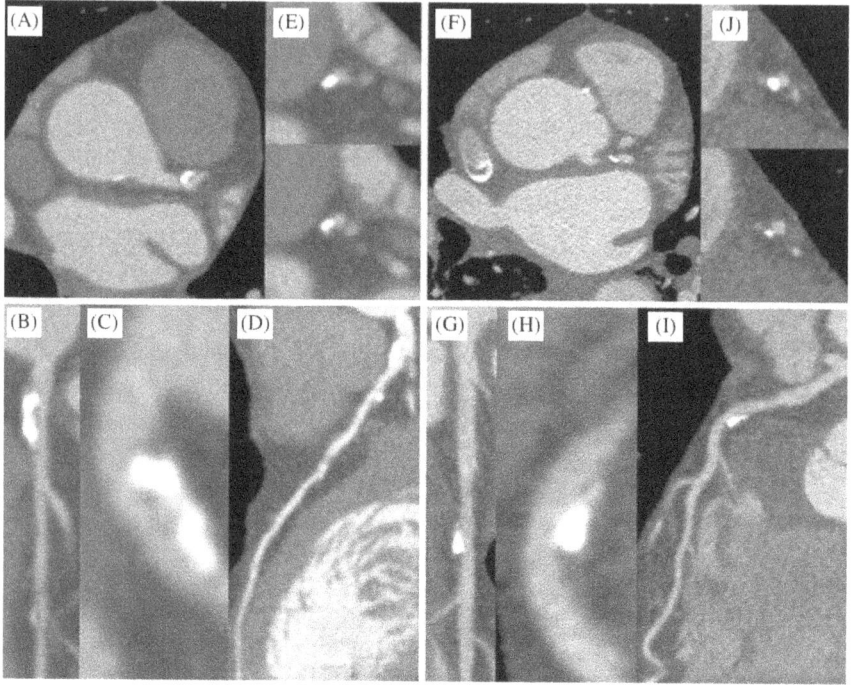

Figure 2.5. High-definition CT vs standard-definition CT in the diagnosis of CAD. A–E: Standard-definition CT in a patient with heart rate of 58 bpm and BMI 24.0 kg/m². F–J: High-definition CT in another patient with HR 58 bpm and BMI 24.0 kg/m². Identical image quality was achieved with these two scanning protocols (1.73 and 1.75 for standard- and high-definition CT scans) and with similar radiation dose (1.66 mSv and 1.51 mSv for standard- and high-definition CT, respectively). 2D axial and curved planar reformatted images show calcified plaques at the left anterior descending coronary artery, with high-definition CT showing superiority in visualizing small and fine details. Reprinted with permission from Kazakauskaite et al.[71]

compromising the specificity and positive predictive value (PPV). The reported specificity of CCTA ranges from 19% to 53% in patients with highly calcified plaques,[72-75] according to the assessment of coronary lumen stenosis. The limitation of standard CCTA can be overcome with improved in-plane spatial resolution of 0.23 mm of high-definition CT, therefore reducing beam hardening and blooming artifacts due to heavy calcification in coronary plaques. Pontone et al. compared the diagnostic value of high spatial resolution (0.23 mm) with standard spatial resolution

(0.625 mm) CCTA in 184 patients at high risk for CAD by using ICA as the reference method.[76] In a segment-based analysis, the specificity and PPV were 98% and 91% for high-definition CCTA, which is significantly higher than the 95% and 80% for standard CCTA. No differences were found in the assessment of non-calcified or mixed plaques between the two groups; however, the overall agreement between CCTA and ICA was significantly improved in the analysis of calcified plaques for high-definition CCTA when compared with the standard CCTA (83%, 91%, 85% and 73% vs 53%, 58%, 51% and 49%, corresponding to all, small, moderate and large calcified plaques, respectively). No significant difference was found in the effective radiation dose between these two groups. High-definition CCTA results in improved overall evaluability, PPV and diagnostic accuracy in heavily calcified plaques, although further research with more evidence is needed to verify these findings.

2.6 Dual-energy CT (DECT)

The main advantages of DECT over single-energy CT are represented by material decomposition by acquiring two image series at the same anatomic location simultaneously with the use of different kVp (80 and 140 kVp) and the elimination of misregistration artifacts. Currently, there are three methods available for simultaneous acquisition of dual-energy images during a single breath-hold: 64-slice or 128-slice DSCT (Definition and Definition Flash, Siemens Medical Systems) with use of two X-ray source and detector pairs, with each source operating at different tube voltage; single source high-definition 64-MDCT (Discovery 750 HD, GE Healthcare) with an X-ray tube capable of rapidly fast kilovolt dynamic switching (from 80 to 140 kVp) between two different energy levels of X-rays from view to view during a single rotation switching; and single X-ray source operating at constant tube voltage with a double-layer detector capable of acquiring the low-energy data from the front or innermost detector layer and high-energy data from the back or outermost detector layer.[77–79]

Conventional CCTA is limited in differentiating different components of plaque characteristics, in particular differentiating lipid-rich from fibrous components within the coronary plaques due to considerable overlap between the lipid-rich and fibrous-rich non-calcified plaques and variable uptake of iodine contrast medium.[80-82] DECT has been shown to potentially overcome such a limitation by providing tissue composition, with increasing reports showing its advantages over single-energy CT.

Scheske *et al.* compared dual-energy with single-energy CT scanners with the aim of determining beam-hardening artifact reduction for evaluation of coronary arteries and myocardium in CCTA.[83] Their results showed significant reduction in beam-hardening artifacts with fast switching DECT, with improvements in signal-to-noise ratio (SNR) and contrast-to-noise (CNR) ratio in the coronary arteries (SNR, 10.83 vs 7.75, CNR, 13.31 vs 9.54, $p < 0.01$) and the myocardium (SNR, 3.02 vs 2.39, CNR, 6.73 vs 5.16, $p < 0.01$), respectively. This is confirmed by other studies which also showed improvement in the detection of myocardial ischemia by suppressing or eliminating beam-hardening artifacts with use of DECT.[84,85] Obaid *et al.* in their *in vivo* and *ex vivo* study demonstrated the improvement of DECT in differentiation of necrotic core and fibrous plaque in the coronary arteries.[86] Dual-energy and single-energy CT images were obtained in 20 patients comprising 138 plaque cross-sections (a total of 1,044 regions of interest) and co-registered with virtual histology intravascular ultrasound (VH-IVUS) for classification of plaque components. Significantly lower overlap of necrotic core and fibrous tissue was found in DECT compared to single-energy CT (Fig. 2.6). Furthermore, DECT showed increased diagnostic accuracy for detection of necrotic core in postmortem arteries, with sensitivity and specificity being 64% and 98%, while the corresponding values for single-energy CT were 50% and 94% (Fig. 2.7). For *in vivo* analysis of necrotic core, DECT has low sensitivity and high specificity of 45% and 91%, but it is still higher than that of single-energy CT, which has values of 39% and 91%.[86]

The incidence of contrast-induced acute kidney injury is associated with contrast-enhanced CT, and this has raised concerns in the literature due to reported evidence in a clinical setting.[87] One of the recommended strategies is to lower contrast medium volume or iodine load while still acquiring diagnostic images. Studies have shown the feasibility of reducing contrast volume or iodine concentration with reduction of radiation dose when compared to the routine contrast volume group in CCTA or CT angiography of aorta.[88-90] In their recent study, Carrascosa *et al.* further confirm the feasibility of this approach in dual-energy CCTA.[91] CCTA

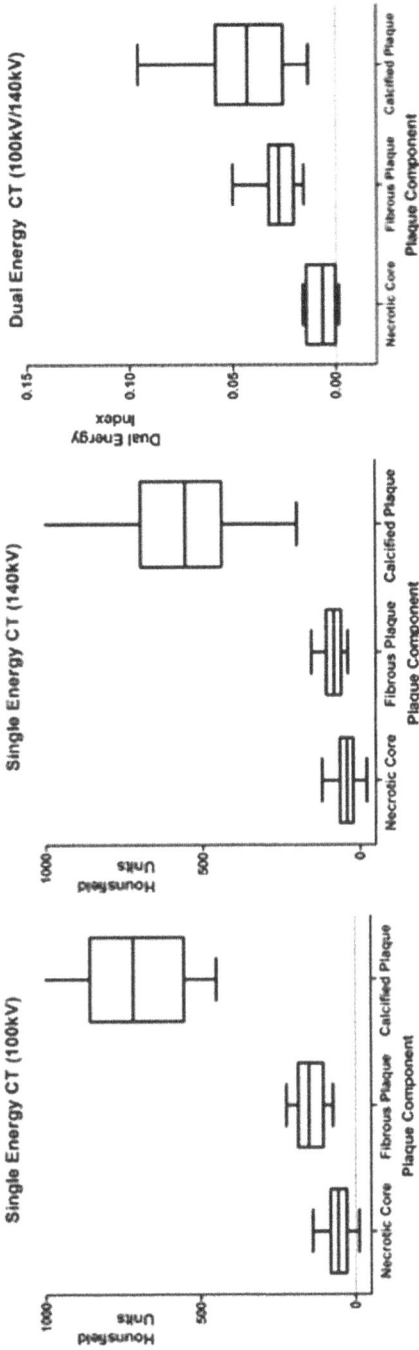

Figure 2.6. Single-energy CT at 100 and 140 kV and dual-energy index of virtual histology-intravascular ultrasound (VH-IVUS)-defined plaque. Box and whisker plots of CT attenuation show marked overlap of necrotic core and fibrous tissues ranges with singe energies 100 and 140 kV. However, dual-energy index ranges for necrotic core did not overlap with any other plaque component. Reprinted with permission under the open access from Obaid et al.[86]

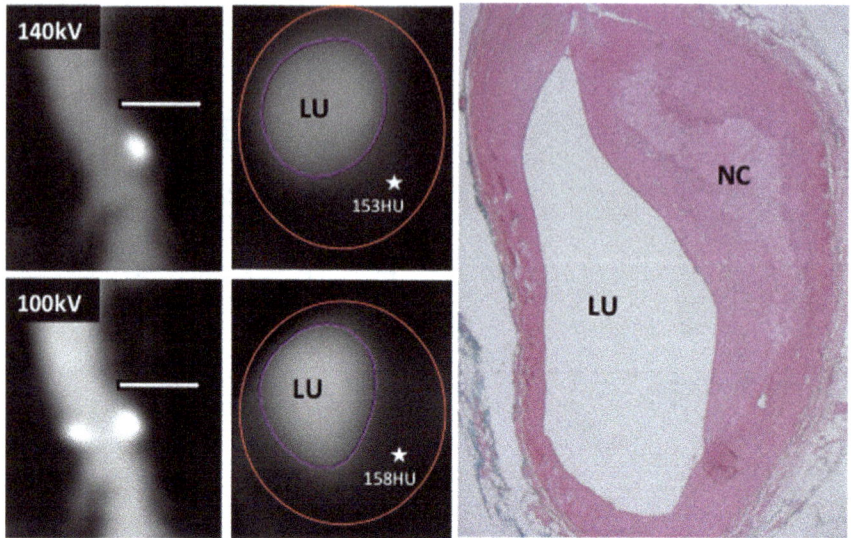

Figure 2.7. Dual-energy CT imaging with postmortem histology. Volume-rendered dual-energy reconstruction (left images) of postmortem coronary artery with attenuation of non-calcified plaque at 100 kV (158 HU) and 140 kV (153 HU) (middle images). These CT attenuation values are above the threshold to classify necrotic core; however, dual-energy index (0.002) correctly identifies the necrotic core confirmed by histology (right images). LU-lumen, NC-necrotic core. Reprinted with permission under the open access from Obaid *et al.*[86]

with half iodine load using DECT imaging was found to have similar image quality scores to single-energy CCTA, with no difference in radiation dose between the two groups. The sensitivity and specificity of CCTA for diagnosis of significant coronary stenosis was similar between the two groups, 84.4% and 87.1%, and 84.4% and 87.1% for dual-energy and single-energy CT, respectively. Despite improved accuracy in DECT in coronary artery and plaque analysis, more studies based on a large cohort of clinical trials are needed to verify these findings.

2.7 Automatic Motion Correction

Although temporal resolution of current CT imaging has significantly improved from 250 ms with early generation of multislice CT scanners to 66 ms with latest CT models, it is still inferior to that of invasive coronary angiography, which is around 10–20 ms. Therefore, heart rate control is still necessary in the majority of patients to ensure acquisition of images with no or fewer artifacts. However, motion artifacts are commonly seen in patients undergoing CCTA scans, especially in patients with high heart rates. Despite effectiveness of beta-blockers to control heart rate, a low heart rate is not always achieved in all patients. In patients with persistently high heart rates, reconstruction algorithms during CCTA are desirable for reduction of motion artifacts.

Automatic motion correction algorithm is a recently developed vendor-specific strategy (Snapshot Freeze, GE Healthcare) or (Adaptive Motion Correction, Toshiba Medical Systems) to improve image quality in patients with high heart rates when compared to conventional CCTA.[92,93] The new algorithm is able to trace the coronary artery path and integrate vessel and velocity from adjacent cardiac phases, thus achieving the goal of motion correction (Fig. 2.8). Leipsic *et al.* in their early study showed

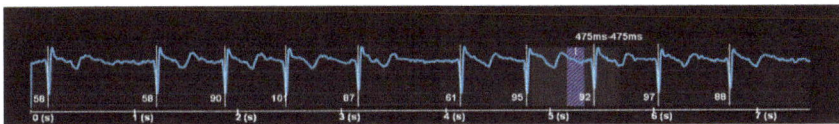

(A)

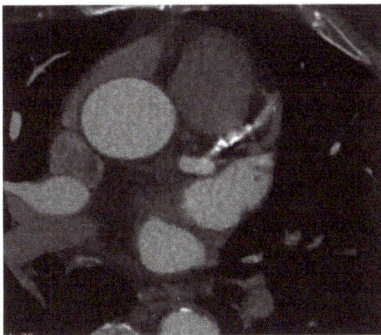 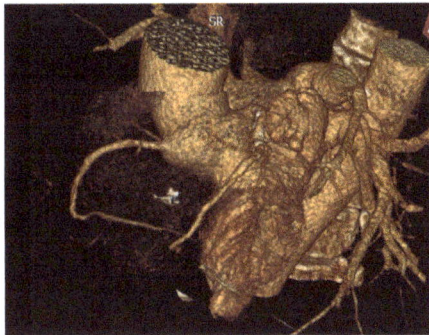

(B)   (C)

Figure 2.8.   Use of automatic motion correction algorithm in CCTA in a 62-year-old male patient. The heart rate is irregular with a minimum of 58 bpm and a maximum of 101 bpm, and heart rate variability of 21. A: electrocardiogram shows the irregular high heart rate in this patient. B: with use of vendor-specific SnapShot Freeze algorithm, coronary artery with calcified plaques is clearly visualized as shown in 2D axial and 3D volume rendering images without being affected by motion artifacts (B and C).

improved image quality and higher interpretability and diagnostic accuracy of CCTA using motion correction reconstructions on a per-segment and per-vessel analysis compared to the standard method, with no significant difference on a per-patient level analysis.[23] The mean heart rate was 71.8 bpm in their study group which consisted of 36 consecutive patients. This is confirmed by some recent studies investigating the effect of automatic correction algorithm in patients with different heart rates.[94–96] According to Lee's study, the use of motion correction in CCTA was associated with significant improvement in sensitivity and specificity on per-segment and per-vessel analysis, with corresponding values increased from 87.3% and 96.9%, and 94.9% and 90.2% with standard CCTA to 94.6% and 99%, and 94.9% and 96.7% with CCTA using motion correction algorithm.[95]

The recently developed GE Revolution scanner is equipped with a 16-cm detector array, thus allowing volumetric single-beat cardiac CT scan with improved image quality, even in patients with high heart rates. Latif *et al.* presented their first experience of using the new CT scanner. In this retrospective study, the authors analyzed images of 439 patients undergoing CCTA performed in a single-beat acquisition within 1 cardiac cycle, irrespective of heart rates. Motion artifacts were corrected by motion correction software in patients with higher heart rate. Diagnostic quality was achieved in patients with higher hear rates (>70 bpm) or large BMI (>30 kg/m^2) through qualitative and quantitative assessments of image quality using the volumetric single-beat new CT scanner.[96]

Fuchs *et al.* have demonstrated significant improvements in image quality and interpretability of CCTA, despite insufficient heart rate control.[93] The authors analyzed 40 patients undergoing CCTA whose heart rates failed to reach the target 63 bpm although beta-blocker was used prior to the CT scan. With use of motion correction algorithm, image quality was significantly improved when compared to the standard reconstruction (3.4 vs 3.0, p < 0.01). Coronary artery interpretability was also improved (88% vs 78%, p < 0.01) in comparison with the standard method. This is confirmed by a latest study showing improvement in image quality and reduction in motion artifacts with the use of motion correction algorithm.[97] Liang and colleagues further confirmed the usefulness of the automatic motion correction algorithm with improved diagnostic performance of CCTA in the diagnosis of CAD.[98] In this recent study consisting of 64 patients with known or suspected CAD with heart rates of 75 bpm, researchers compared diagnostic value of CCTA in images using automatic motion correction algorithm compared to the standard method with ICA as the reference method. On per-segment assessment, sensitivity, specificity, PPV and negative predictive value were 93.7%, 85.1%, 50.2% and 98.5% for standard CCTA and 91.9%, 95.8%, 77.9% and 98.7% for CCTA with the use of motion correction algorithm; on per-artery assessment, these values were 98.7%, 74%, 62.9% and 99.2% for standard CCTA and 96.2%, 94.4%, 77.9% and 98.7% for CCTA with the use of motion correction algorithm; and on per-patient assessment, these values were 100%, 14.3%, 70.5% and 100% for standard CCTA and 100%, 85.7%, 93.5% and 100% for CCTA using motion correction algorithm. The area under receiver operating characteristics curve was also significantly improved with corresponding value being 0.91 vs 0.60 (p < 0.01) for CCTA with and without use of motion correction algorithm.[98] Further research with inclusion of large cohort and multicenter studies is needed to validate the diagnostic accuracy of using motion correction algorithm in CCTA for the diagnosis of significant coronary stenosis.

2.8 Summary

Various current and new imaging techniques have been developed in recent years to improve diagnostic value of CCTA with generation of acceptable images but with much lower radiation dose. These techniques, which include prospective ECG-triggering, high-pitch helical CT scan, IR algorithms, high-definition CT, automatic tube potential modulation, DECT and automatic motion correction or reconstruction, have not only significantly lowered the radiation dose but have also improved overall assessment of coronary artery stenosis and image interpretability, therefore improving diagnostic performance. Understanding these technical approaches and appropriate use of these imaging techniques plays an important role in maximizing the clinical applications of CCTA for accurate diagnosis of CAD and improvement of patient care and clinical management.

References

1. Sun Z, Jiang W. (2006) Diagnostic value of multislice CT angiography in coronary artery disease: a meta-analysis. *Eur J Radiol* **60**: 279–286.

2. Sun Z, Lin CH, Davidson R, Dong C, Liao Y. (2008) Diagnostic value of 64-slice CT angiography in coronary artery disease: a systematic review. *Eur J Radiol* **67**: 78–84.

3. Vanhoenacker P, Heijenbrok-Kal M, Van Heste R *et al.* (2007) Diagnostic performance of multidetector CT angiography for assessment of coronary artery disease: meta-analysis. *Radiology* **244**: 419–442.

4. Abdulla J, Abildstrom Z, Gotzsche O, Christensen E, Kober L, Torp-Pedersen C. (2007) 64-multislice detector computed tomography coronary angiography as potential alternative to conventional coronary angiography: a systematic review and meta-analysis. *Eur Heart J* **28**: 3042–3050.

5. Stein PD, Yaekoub AY, Matta F, Sostman HD. (2008) 64-slice CT for diagnosis of coronary artery disease: a systematic review. *Am J Med* **121**: 715–725.

6. Mowatt G, Cook JA, Hillis GS *et al.* (2008) 64-slice computed tomography angiography in the diagnosis and assessment of coronary artery disease: systematic review and meta-analysis. *Heart* **94**: 1386–1393.

7. Miller JM, Rochitte CE, Dewey M *et al.* (2008) Diagnostic performance of coronary angiography by 64-row CT. *N Engl J Med* **359**: 2324–2336.

8. Voros S. (2009) What are the potential advantages and disadvantages of volumetric CT scanning? *J Cardiovasc Comput Tomogr* **3**: 67–70.

9. Salavati A, Radmanesh F, Heidari K, Dwamena BA, Kelly AM, Cronin P. (2012) Dual-source computed tomography angiography for diagnosis and assessment of coronary artery disease: systematic review and meta-analysis. *J Cardiovasc Comput Tomogr* **6**: 78–90.

10. van Ballmoos MW, Haring B, Juillerat P, Alkadhi H. (2011) Meta-analysis: diagnostic performance of low-radiation-dose coronary computed tomography angiography. *Ann Intern Med* **154**: 413–420.

11. Sun Z, Ng KH. (2012) Diagnostic value of coronary CT angiography with prospective ECG-gating in the diagnosis of coronary artery disease: a systematic review and meta-analysis. *Int J Cardiovasc Imaging* **28**: 2109–2119.

12. Sun Z, Ng KH. (2012) Prospective versus retrospective ECG-gated multislice CT coronary angiography: a systematic review of radiation dose and diagnostic accuracy. *Eur J Radiol* **81**: e94–e100.

13. Sabarudin A, Sun Z, Ng KH. (2013) Coronary CT angiography with prospective ECG-triggering: a systematic review of image quality and radiation dose. *Singapore Med J* **54**: 15–23.

14. Machida H, Tanaka I, Fukui R *et al.* (2015) Current and novel imaging techniques in coronary CT. *Radiographics* **356**: 991–1010.

15. Puchner SB, Ferencik M, Maurovich-Horvat P *et al.* (2015) Iterative image reconstruction algorithms in coronary CT angiography improve the detection of lipid-core plaque — a comparison with histology. *Eur Radiol* **25**: 15–23.

16. Oda S, Weissman G, Vembar M, Weigold WG. (2014) Iterative model reconstruction: improved image quality of low-tube voltage prospective ECG-gated coronary CT angiography images at 256-slice CT. *Eur J Radiol* **83**: 1408–1415.

17. Szilveszter B, Celeng C, Maurovich-Horvat P. (2015) Plaque assessment by coronary CT. *Int J Cardiovasc Imaging* **32**: 161–172.

18. Chung HW, Ko SM, Hwang HK, So Y, Yi JG, Lee EJ. (2017) Diagnostic performance of coronary CT angiography, stress dual-energy CT perfusion, and stress perfusion single-photon emission computed tomography for coronary artery disease: Comparison with combined invasive coronary angiography and stress perfusion cardiac MRI. *Korean J Radiol* **18**(3): 476–486.

19. Yang WJ, Zhang H, Xiao H *et al.* (2012) High-definition computed tomography for coronary artery stents imaging compared with standard-definition 64-row multidetector computed tomography: an initial in vivo study. *J Comput Assist Tomogr* **36**(3): 295–300.

20. Min JK, Swaminathan RV, Vass M, Gallagher S, Weinsaft JW. (2009) High-definition multidetector computed tomography for evaluation of coronary artery stents: comparison to standard-definition 64-detector row computed tomography. *J Cardiovasc Comput Tomogr* **3**(4): 246–251.

21. Vliegenthart R, Pelgrim GJ, Ebersberger U, Rowe GW, Oudkerk M, Schoepf UJ. (2012) Dual-energy CT of the heart. *AJR Am J Roentgenol* **199**(5 Suppl): S54–63.

22. Machida H, Lin XZ, Fukui R *et al.* (2015) Influence of the motion correction algorithm on the quality and interpretability of single-source 64-detector coronary CT angiography among patients grouped by heart rate. *Jpn J Radiol* **33**(2): 84–93.

23. Leipsic J, Labounty TM, Hague CJ *et al.* (2012) Effect of a novel vendor-specific motion-correction algorithm on image quality and diagnostic accuracy in persons undergoing coronary CT angiography without rate-control medications. *J Cardiovasc Comput Tomogr* **6**(3): 164–171.

24. Sun Z, Choo GH, Ng KH. (2012) Coronary CT angiography: current status and continuing challenges. *Br J Radiol* **85**: 495–510.

25. Lu B, Lu JG, Sun ML *et al.* (2011) Comparison of diagnostic accuracy and radiation dose between prospective triggering and retrospective gated coronary angiography by dual-source computed tomography. *Am J Cardiol* **107**: 1278–1284.

26. Maruyama T, Takada M, Hasuike T, Yoshikawa A, Namimatsu E, Yoshizumi T. (2008) Radiation dose reduction and coronary assessability of prospective electrocardiogram-gated computed tomography coronary angiography: comparison with retrospective electrocardiogram-gated helical scan. *J Am Coll Cardiol* **52**: 1450–1455.

27. Stolzmann P, Leschka S, Scheffel H *et al.* (2008) Dual-source CT in step-and-shoot mode: non-invasive coronary angiography with low radiation dose. *Radiology* **249**: 71–80.

28. Freeman A, Learner R, Eggleton S, Lambros J, Friedman D. (2011) Marked reduction of effective radiation dose in patients undergoing CT coronary angiography using prospective ECG gating. *Heart Lung Circ* **20**: 512–516.

29. Sabarudin A, Sun Z, Yusof AK. (2013) Coronary CT angiography with single-source and dual-source CT: comparison of image quality and radiation dose between prospective ECG-triggered and retrospective ECG-gated protocols. *Int J Cardiol* **168**: 746–753.

30. Pontone G, Andreini D, Bartorelli A *et al.* (2009) Diagnostic accuracy of coronary computed tomography angiography: a comparison between prospective and retrospective electrocardiogram triggering. *J Am Coll Cardiol* **54**: 346–355.

31. Xu L, Yang L, Zhang Z *et al.* (2010) Low-dose adaptive sequential scan for dual-source CT coronary angiography in patients with high heart rate: comparison with retrospective ECG-gating. *Eur J Radiol* **76**: 183–187.

32. Yang L, Zhou T, Zhang R *et al.* (2014) Meta-analysis: diagnostic accuracy of coronary CT angiography with prospective ECG gating based on step-and-shoot, flash and volume modes for detection of coronary artery disease. *Eur Radiol* **24**: 2345–2352.

33. Menke J, Unterberg-Buchwald C, Staab W *et al.* (2013) Head-to-head comparison of prospectively triggered vs retrospectively gated coronary computed tomography angiography: meta-analysis of diagnostic accuracy, image quality, and radiation dose. *Am Heart J* **165**: 154–163.

34. Sun Z. (2012) Coronary CT angiography with prospective ECG-triggering: an effective alternative to invasive coronary angiography. *Cardiovasc Diag Ther* **2**: 28–37.

35. Bogaard K, van der Zant FM, Knol RJ *et al.* (2015) High-pitch prospective ECG-triggered helical coronary computed tomography angiography in clinical practice: image quality and radiation dose. *Int J Cardiovasc Imaging* **31**: 125–133.

36. Sun M, Lu B, Wu R, *et al.* (2011) Diagnostic accuracy of dual-source CT coronary angiography with prospective ECG-triggering on different heart rate patients. *Eur Radiol* **21**: 1635–1642.

37. Park CH, Lee J, Oh C, Han KH, Kim TH (2015) The feasibility of sub-millisievert coronary CT angiography with low tube voltage, prospective ECG gating, and a knowledge-based iterative model reconstruction algorithm. *Int J Cardiovasc Imaging* **31**(Suppl 2): 179–203.

38. Hoe J, Toh KH. (2009) First experience with 320-row multidetector CT coronary angiography scanning with prospective electrocardiogram gating to reduce radiation dose. *J Cardiovasc Comput Tomogr* **3**: 257–261.

39. Achenbach S, Marwan M, Ropers D *et al.* (2010) Coronary computed tomography angiography with a consistent dose below 1 mSv using prospectively electrocardiogram-triggered high-pitch spiral acquisition. *Eur Heart J* **31**: 340–346.

40. Lell M, Marvan M, Schepis T *et al.* (2009) Prospectively ECG-triggered high-pitch spiral acquisition for coronary CT angiography using dual source CT: technique and initial experience. *Eur Radiol* **19**: 2576–2583.

41. Alkadhi H, Stolzmann P, Desbiolles L *et al.* (2010) Low-dose, 128-slice, dual-source CT coronary angiography: accuracy and radiation dose of the high-pitch and the step-and-shoot mode. *Heart* **96**: 933–938.

42. Yin WH, Lu B, Hou ZH *et al.* (2013) Detection of coronary artery stenosis with sub-milliSievert radiation dose by prospectively ECG-triggered high-pitch spiral CT angiography and iterative reconstruction. *Eur Radiol* **23**: 2927–2933.

43. Gordic S, Husarik DB, Desbiolles L *et al.* (2014) High-pitch coronary CT angiography with third generation dual-source CT: limits of heart rate. *Int J Cardiovasc Imaging* **30**: 1173–1179.

44. Feng R, Mao J, Liu X, Zhao Y, Tong J, Zhang L. (2017) High-pitch coronary computed tomographic angiography using the third-generation dual-source computed tomography: Initial Experience in patients with high heart rate. J Comput Assist Tomogr Sep 20. doi: 10.1097/RCT.0000000000000678. [Epub ahead of print]

45. Hausleiter J, Martinoff S, Hadamitzky M *et al.* (2010) Image quality and radiation exposure with a low tube voltage protocol for coronary CT angiography results of the PROTECTION II Trial. *JACC Cardiovasc Imaging* **3**: 1113–1123.

46. Leschka S, Stolzmann P, Schmid FT *et al.* (2008) Low kilovoltage cardiac dual-source CT: Attenuation, noise, and radiation dose. *Eur Radiol* **18**: 1809–1817.

47. Feuchtner GM, Jodocy D, Klauser A *et al.* (2010) Radiation dose reduction by using 100-kV tube voltage in cardiac 64-slice computed tomography: a comparative study. *Eur J Radiol* **75**: e51–e56.

48. Blankstein R, Bolen MA, Pale R *et al.* (2011) Use of 100 kV versus 120 kV in cardiac dual source computed tomography: effect on radiation dose and image quality. *Int J Cardiovasc Imaging* **27**: 579–586.

49. Pflederer T, Jakstat J, Marwan M *et al.* (2010) Radiation exposure and image quality in staged low-dose protocols for coronary dual-source CT angiography: a randomized comparison. *Eur Radiol* **20**: 1197–1206.

50. Halliburton SS, Abbara S, Chen MY *et al.* (2011) SCCT guidelines on radiation dose and dose-optimization strategies in cardiovascular CT. *J Cardiovasc Comput Tomogr* **5**: 198–224.

51. Raff GL, Chinnaiyan KM, Cury RC *et al.* (2014) SCCT guidelines on the use of coronary computed tomographic angiography for patients presenting with acute chest pain to the emergency department: a report of the Society of Cardiovascular Computed Tomography Guidelines Committee. *J Cardiovasc Comput Tomogr* **8**: 254–271.

52. Ghoshhajra BB, Engel LC, Major GP *et al.* (2011) Direct chest area measurement: a potential anthropometric replacement for BMI to inform cardiac CT dose parameters? *J Cardiovasc Comput Tomogr* **5**: 240–246.

53. Ghoshhajra BB, Engel LC, Karolyi M *et al.* (2013) Cardiac computed tomography angiography with automatic tube potential selection: effects on radiation dose and image quality. *J Thorac Imaging* **28**: 40–48.

54. Layritz C, Muschiol G, Flohr T *et al.* (2013) Automated attenuation-based selection of tube voltage and tube current for coronary CT angiography: reduction of radiation exposure versus BMI-based strategy with an expert investigator. *J Cardiovasc Comput Tomogr* **7**: 303–310.

55. Iyama Y, Nakaura T, Kidoh M *et al.* (2016) Submillisievert radiation dose Coronary CT angiography: clinical impact of the knowledge-based iterative model reconstruction. *Acad Radiol* **23**: 1391–1401.

56. Benz DC, Fuchs TA, Gräni C *et al.* (2017) Head-to-head comparison of adaptive statistical and model based iterative reconstruction algorithms for submillisievert coronary CT angiography. doi: 10.1093/ehjci/jex008.

57. den Harder AM, Wolterink JM, J *et al.* (2016) Submillisievert coronary calcium quantification using model-based iterative reconstruction: A within-patient analysis. *Eur J Radiol* **85**: 2152–2159.

58. Leipsic J, Heilbron BG, Hague C. (2012) Iterative reconstruction for coronary CT angiography: finding its way. *Int J Cardiovasc Imaging* **28**: 613–620.

59. Leipsic J, Labounty TM, Heilbron B *et al.* (2010) Estimated radiation dose reduction using adaptive statistical iterative reconstruction in coronary CT angiography: the ERASIR study. *AJR Am J Roentgenol* **195**(3): 655–660.

60. Tumur O, Soon K, Mykytowycz M. (2013) New scanning technique using adaptive statistical iterative reconstruction (ASIR) significantly reduced the radiation dose of cardiac CT. *J Med Imaging Radiat Oncol* **57**: 292–296.

61. Chen MY, Shanbhag SM, Arai AE. (2013) Submillisievert median radiation dose for coronary angiography with a second-generation 320-detector row CT scanner in 107 consecutive patients. *Radiology* **267**: 76–85.

62. Hell MM, Bittner D, Schuhbaek A *et al.* (2014) Prospectively ECG-triggered high-pitch coronary angiography with third-generation dual-source CT at 70 kVp tube voltage: feasibility, image quality, radiation dose, and effect of iterative reconstruction. *J Cardiovasc Comput Tomogr* **8**: 418–425.

63. Meyer M, Haubenreisser H, Schoepf UJ *et al.* (2014) Closing in on the K edge: coronary CT angiography at 100, 80, and 70 kV-initial comparison of a second- versus a third-generation dual-source CT system. *Radiology* **272**: 373–382.

64. Stehli J, Fuschs TA, Bull S *et al.* (2014) Accuracy of coronary CT angiography using a submillisievert fraction of radiation exposure: comparison with invasive coronary angiography. *J Am Coll Cardiol* **64**: 772–780.

65. Schuhnaeck A, Achenbach S, Layritz C *et al.* (2013) Image quality of ultra-low radiation exposure coronary CT angiography with an effective dose <0.1 mSv using high-pitch spiral acquisition and raw data-based iterative reconstruction. *Eur Radiol* **23**: 597–606.

66. Den Harder AM, Willemink MJ, De Ruiter QM *et al.* (2016) Dose reduction with iterative reconstruction for coronary CT angiography: a systematic review and meta-analysis. *Br J Radiol* **89**: 20150068.

67. Alkadhi H, Leschka S. (2011) Radiation dose of cardiac computed tomography — what has been achieved and what needs to be done. *Eur J Radiol* **21**: 505–509.

68. Liang J, Wang H, Xu L *et al.* (2017) Diagnostic performance of 256-row detector coronary CT angiography in patients with high heart rates within a single cardiac cycle: a preliminary study. *Clin Radiol* **72**: 694.e7–694.e14.

69. Yang WJ, Zhang H, Xiao H *et al.* (2012) High-definition computed tomography for coronary artery stents imaging compared with standard-definition 64-row multidetector computed tomography: an initial in vivo study. *J Comput Assist Tomogr* **36**: 295–300.

70. Min JK, Swaminathan RV, Vass M, Gallagher S, Weinsaft JW. (2009) High-definition multidetector computed tomography for evaluation of coronary artery stents: comparison to standard-definition 64-detector row computed tomography. *J Cardiovasc Comput Tomogr* **3**: 246–251.

71. Kazakauskaite E, Husmann L, Stehli J *et al.* (2013) Image quality in low-dose coronary computed tomography angiography with a new high-definition CT scanner. *Int J Cardiovasc Imaging* **29**: 471–477.

72. Park MJ, Jung JI, Choi YS *et al.* (2011) Coronary CT angiography in patients with high calcium score: evaluation of plaque characteristics and diagnostic accuracy. *Int J Cardiovasc Imaging* **27**: 43–51.

73. Sun Z, Ng C. (2015) High calcium scores in coronary CT angiography: effects of image post-processing on visualization and measurement of coronary lumen diameter. *J Med Imaging Health Inf* **5**: 110–116.

74. Chen CC, Chen CC, Hsieh IC *et al.* (2011) The effect of calcium score on the diagnostic accuracy of coronary computed tomography angiography. *Int J Cardiovasc Imaging* **Suppl 1**: 37–42.

75. Meng L, Cui L, Cheng Y *et al.* (2009) Effect of heart rate and coronary calcification on the diagnostic accuracy of the dual-source CT coronary angiography in patients with suspected coronary artery disease. *Korean J Radiol* **10**: 347–354.

76. Pontone G, Bertella E, Mushtaq S *et al.* (2014) Coronary artery disease: diagnostic accuracy of CT coronary angiography — a comparison of high and standard spatial resolution scanning. *Radiology* **271**: 688–694.

77. Karcaaltincaba M, Aktas A. (2011) Dual-energy CT revisited with multidetector CT: review of principles and clinical applications. *Diagn Interv Radiol* **17**: 181–194.

78. Danad I, Fayad ZA, Willemink MJ, Min JK. (2015) New applications of cardiac computed tomography: dual-energy, spectral, and molecular CT imaging. *JACC Cardiovasc Imaging* **8**: 710–723.

79. McCoullough CH, Leng S, Yu L, Fletcher JG. (2015) Dual- and multi-energy CT: principles, technical approaches and clinical applications. *Radiology* **276**: 637–653.

80. Petranovic M, Soni A, Bezzera H *et al.* (2009) Assessment of nonstenotic coronary lesions by 64-slice multidetector computed tomography in comparison to intravascular ultrasound: evaluation of nonculprit coronary lesions. *J Cardiovasc Comput Tomogr* **3**: 24–31.

81. Leber AW, Knez A, Becker A *et al.* (2004) Accuracy of multidetector spiral computed tomography in identifying and differentiating the composition of coronary atherosclerotic plaques: a comparative study with intracoronary ultrasound. *J Am Coll Cardiol* **43**: 1241–1247.

82. Pohle K, Achenbach S, Macneill B *et al.* (2007) Characterization of non-calcified coronary atherosclerotic plaque by multi-detector row CT: comparison to IVUS. *Atherosclerosis* **190**: 174–180.

83. Scheske JA, O'Brien JM, Earls JP *et al.* (2013) Coronary artery imaging with single-source rapid kilovolt peak-switching dual-energy CT. *Radiology* **268**: 702–709.

84. So A, Hsieh J, Narayanan S *et al.* (2012) Dual-energy CT and its potential use for quantitative myocardial CT perfusion. *J Cardiovasc Comput Tomogr* **6**: 308–317.

85. Yamada M, Jinzaki M, Kuribayashi S, Imanishi N, Funato K, Aiso S. (2012) Beam-hardening correction for virtual monochromatic imaging of myocardial perfusion via fast-switching dual-kVp 64-slice computed tomography: a pilot study using a human heart specimen. *Circ J* **76**: 1799–1801.

86. Obaid DR, Calvert PA, Gopalan D *et al.* (2014) Dual-energy computed tomography imaging to determine atherosclerotic plaque composition: a prospective study with tissue validation. *J Cardiovasc Comput Tomogr* **8**: 230–237.

87. Mitchell AM, Jones AE, Tumlin JA, Kline JA. (2010) Incidence of contrast-induced nephropathy after contrast-enhanced computed tomography in the outpatient setting. *Clin J Am Soc Nephrol: CJASN* **5**: 4–9.

88. Shen Y, Fan Z, Sun Z *et al.* (2015) High pitch dual-source whole aorta CT angiography in the detection of coronary arteries: a feasibility study of using iodixanol 270 and 100 kVp with iterative reconstruction. *J Med Imaging Health Inf* **5**: 117–125.

89. Zheng M, Liu Y, Wei M, Wu Y, Zhao H, Li J. (2014) Low concentration contrast medium for dual-source computed tomography coronary angiography by a combination of iterative reconstruction and low-tube-voltage technique. *Eur J Radiol* **83**: e92–e99.

90. Shen Y, Sun Z, Xu L *et al.* (2015) High-pitch, low-voltage and low-iodine concentration CT angiography of aorta: assessment of image quality and radiation dose with iterative reconstruction. *Plos One* **10**: e0117469.

91. Carrascosa P, Leipsic JA, Capunay C *et al.* (2015) Monochromatic image reconstruction by dual energy imaging allows half iodine load computed coronary angiography. *Eur J Radiol* **84**: 1915–1920.

92. Bischoff B, Geyer LL, Reiser MF, Mueller Lisse UG. (2015) Improved image quality of coronary CT angiography using automatic motion correction. *Arch Cardiovasc Imaging* **3**: e28932.

93. Fuchs TA, Stehli J, Dougoud S *et al.* (2014) Impact of a new motion-correction algorithm on image quality of low-dose coronary CT angiography in patients with insufficient heart rate control. *Acad Radiol* **21**: 312–317.

94. Li Q, Li P, Su Z *et al.* (2014) Effect of a novel motion correction algorithm (SSF) on the image quality of coronary CTA with intermediate heart rates: segment-based and vessel-based analyses. *Eur J Radiol* **83**: 2024–2032.

95. Lee H, Kim JA, Lee JS *et al.* (2014) Impact of a vendor-specific motion-correction algorithm on image quality, interpretability, and diagnostic performance of daily routine coronary CT angiography: influence of heart rate on the effect of motion-correction. *Int J Cardiovasc Imaging* **30**: 1603–1612.

96. Latif MA, Sanchez FW, Sayegh K *et al.* (2016) Volumetric single-beat coronary computed tomography angiography: relationship of image quality, heart rate, and body mass index. Initial patient experience with a new computed tomography scanner. *J Comput Assist Tomogr* **40**: 763–772.

97. Sheta HM, Egstrup K, Husic M, Heinsen LJ, Nieman K, Lambrechtsen J. (2017) Impact of a motion correction algorithm on image quality in patients undergoing CT angiography: a randomized controlled trial. *Clin Imaging* **42**: 1–6.

98. Liang J, Wang H, Xu L *et al.* (2017) Impact of SSF on diagnostic performance of coronary computed tomography angiography within 1 heart beat in patients with high heart rate using a 256-row detector computed tomography. *J Comput Assist Tomogr* doi: 10.1097/RCT.0000000000000641.

3 Coronary CT Angiography: 2D and 3D Characterization of Coronary Plaques

Table of Contents

Abstract

Coronary computed tomography angiography (CCTA) has high diagnostic value in the detection and quantitative analysis of coronary plaques. 2D and 3D reconstructions allow accurate assessment of plaque characteristics by CCTA. In addition, development of image postprocessing techniques enables quantitative analysis of plaques with CCTA, thus providing valuable information for prediction of major adverse cardiac events. The aim of this chapter is to provide an overview of CCTA-generated various 2D and 3D visualizations, with a focus on quantitative assessment of plaque features. Recent research on automatic plaque quantification is also discussed.

Keywords: assessment, coronary CT angiography, coronary plaque, quantification, three-dimensional reconstruction.

3.1 Introduction

Coronary computed tomography angiography (CCTA) is a reliable imaging modality for assessment of coronary artery disease (CAD) due to its capability of detecting the coronary lumen and wall changes with high accuracy.[1–3] The state-of-the-art CT scanners combined with image reconstruction methods allow for acquisition of images with excellent quality, thus, enabling detection and characterization of coronary plaques with high accuracy.[4–6]

CT characterization of plaque morphology has potential clinical significance, since autopsy studies in coronary death have indicated that the site of coronary thrombosis is often associated with plaque rupture at sites with a thin fibrous plaque cap and a large lipid core.[7–9] Intravascular ultrasound (IVUS) is widely recognized as the gold standard for quantitative analysis of plaque components as it allows assessment of cross-sectional areas of the coronary artery which are closely associated with the hemodynamic significance of coronary stenosis.[10–12] Although IVUS is the standard reference for the assessment of coronary plaque composition and progression in clinical studies, it is an invasive procedure which is not routinely performed in daily clinical practice. CCTA has been increasingly used in the evaluation of coronary plaque characteristics, including plaque compositions and differentiation of stable from unstable or high-risk plaques in addition to lumen stenosis. The introduction of semi- or automatic plaque quantification has further advanced both diagnostic and prognostic values of CCTA when compared to traditional risk factors.[13,14] This chapter summarizes the CCTA plaque characterization and assessment, with a focus on plaque features and corresponding CCTA appearances as shown on 2D and 3D reconstructions. Recent developments in automatic quantification of coronary plaques are also discussed.

3.2 2D and 3D Image Reconstructions

CCTA in imaging CAD is complemented by a number of 2D and 3D reconstructed visualizations, including multiplanar reformation (MPR)/ curved planar reformation (CVR), maximum-intensity projection (MIP), volume rendering (VR), and virtual intravascular endoscopy

(VIE). Although 2D axial CT images still remain as the initial visualization tool in most situations, 2D and 3D reconstructed visualizations provide additional information for identification and characterization of coronary plaques which plays an important role in assisting accurate diagnosis.

With 64- or more slice CT scanners becoming widely available, a voxel size of $0.35 \times 0.35 \times 0.35$ mm^3 can be achieved in all three dimensions (x, y and z direction) in axial CT images, thus, enabling excellent visualization of the cardiovascular structures, including the tiny coronary arteries (Fig. 3.1). Image quality of original source data determines the 2D or 3D reconstructed visualizations.

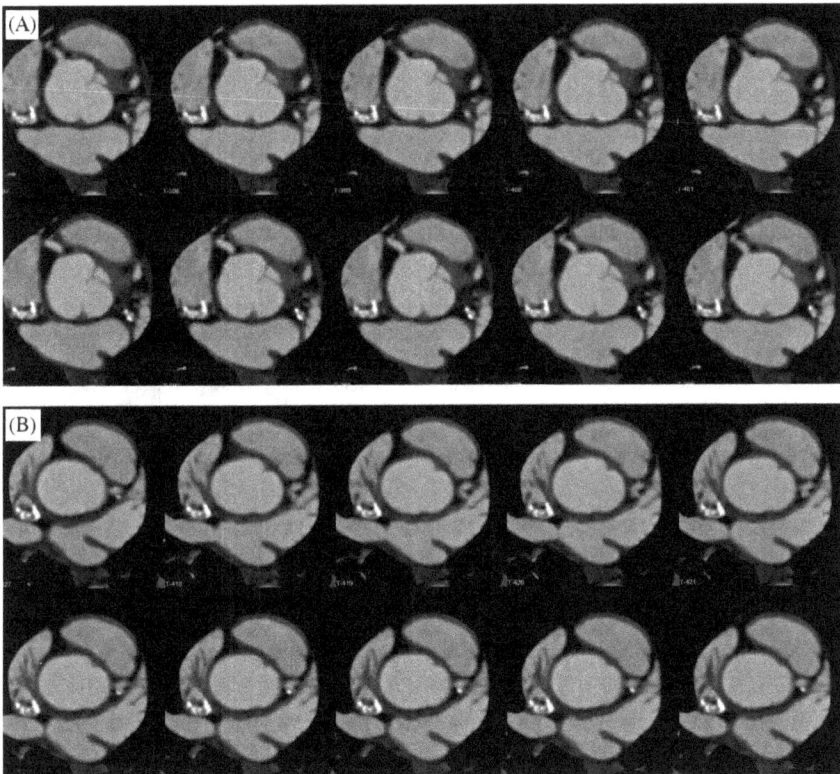

Figure 3.1. A series of 2D axial coronary CT angiographic images acquired with 64-slice CT scanner show the normal right coronary artery (A) and calcified plaque at the left circumflex artery (B).

MPR is most commonly used in CT angiography as it improves understanding of the relationship among complex anatomical structures by presenting images in coronal, sagittal or oblique sections. However, conventional MPR views have limited role in cardiac imaging since coronary arteries show complex course without following a straight path along the myocardium. In contrast, CPR also called CVR is the most useful visualization tool for cardiac CT as MPR views are generated along the curved planes instead of straight planes. CVR enables the capture of the course of tortuous coronary arteries along their entire length in a single image (Fig. 3.2), and it has become a routine visualization tool for demonstration of the entire coronary artery tree in CCTA.

MIP is the most useful reconstructed visualization in CT angiography as it allows for generation of angiographic-like images but in a less-invasive approach when compared to invasive angiography. MIP is less commonly used in imaging coronary arteries than the non-cardiac CT angiography. MIP images lack depth information as this reconstruction tool is a 2D representation of 3D volume data, thus, limiting its value in visualization of complex anatomy such as coronary arteries. Thin-slap MIPs are used to overcome this limitation by generating planes in parallel

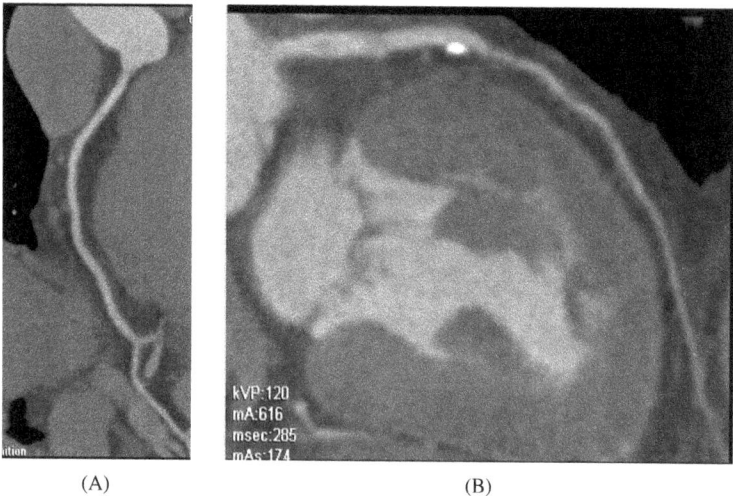

(A)   (B)

Figure 3.2. (A) curved planar reformatted (CVR) shows a normal right coronary artery with excellent visualization of the entire coronary artery tree. (B) CVR shows a calcified plaque at proximal segment of left anterior descending (LAD) coronary artery.

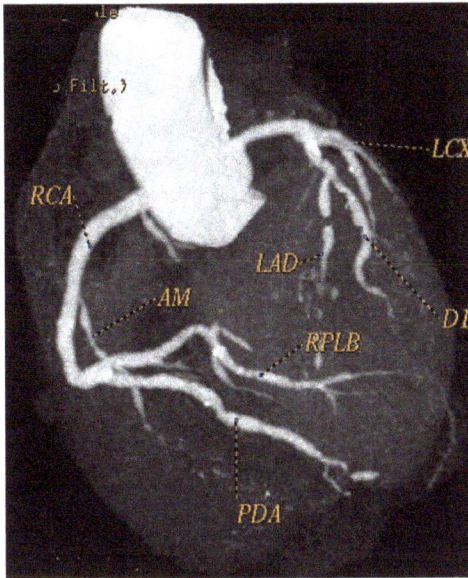

Figure 3.3. The slab MIP shows coronary artery and side branches. AM — acute marginal branch, D1 — diagonal branch, LAD — left anterior descending, LCx — left circumflex, PDA — posterior descending artery, RCA — right coronary artery, RPLB — right posterolateral branch.

to a line connecting the coronary artery to show the course of coronary arteries (Fig. 3.3).

3D VR is commonly used in imaging coronary arteries due to its capability of demonstrating 3D relationship between different structures in a single image. A voxel-based intensity histogram is generated, and several parameters such as color, brightness and opacity are assigned to each voxel according to its Hounsfield unit (HU) value. This provides more meaningful images, in particular, when assessing the coronary arteries in relation to the location of plaques and degree of stenosis (Fig. 3.4).

A new and novel 3D VR visualization tool has been developed very recently, called cinematic rendering that enhances visualization of anatomical detail and pathology.[15,16] Cinematic rendering produces photorealistic images, enabling more accurate depiction of pathology in relation to the anatomical structures than the conventional 3D VR technique. This

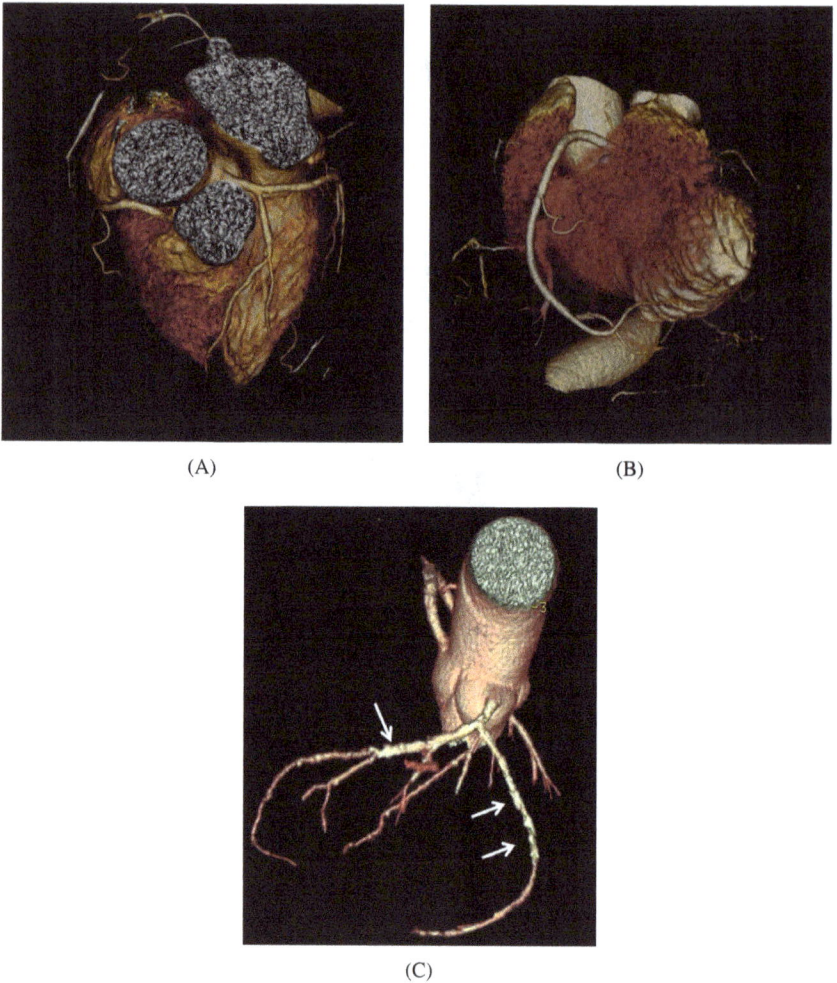

(A)

(B)

(C)

Figure 3.4. 3D VR shows normal left coronary artery (A) and right coronary artery (B). 3D VR in another patient shows coronary plaques (arrows) present at the LAD and left circumflex arteries with irregular coronary lumen changes (C).

new visualization algorithm has not yet been clinically approved. Further studies are needed to determine its diagnostic accuracy and how cinematic imaging is incorporated in clinical practice.

VIE represents another 3D visualization tool, but offers unique intra-vascular views of the artery wall and any other pathological changes such

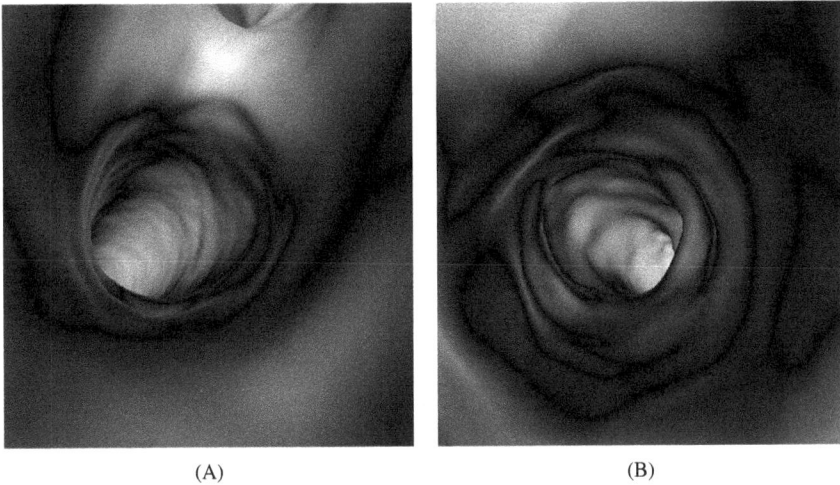

(A)   (B)

Figure 3.5. VIE reveals intraluminal views of left coronary ostium (A) and right coronary ostium (B) with smooth appearance.

as plaque position, appearances and degree of lumen stenosis.[17–20] Traditional 2D or 3D visualizations provide external views of the arterial system and abnormal changes, while VIE offers inside views of the coronary artery and plaque appearances, thus providing additional information to the existing tools. Figure 3.5 is an example of VIE visualization of normal coronary lumen, while Figure 3.6 shows coronary plaques at the LAD artery in a patient diagnosed with CAD.

3.3 Characterization of Coronary Plaques

Coronary plaques are commonly characterized into three types according to the CT attenuation: calcified plaque, non-calcified and mixed plaques.[21–23] Calcified plaque is defined as one with 50% or greater calcium present within the lesions and CT density greater than 220 HU. Thus, a calcified lesion refers to any structure that can be visualized separately from the contrast-enhanced coronary lumen. Figure 3.7 shows calcified plaques in the LAD coronary artery. When lesions have less than 50% calcium but CT attenuation is ≥130 HU, they are defined as mixed plaques. Figure 3.8 is an example of a mixed plaque at the LAD coronary artery.

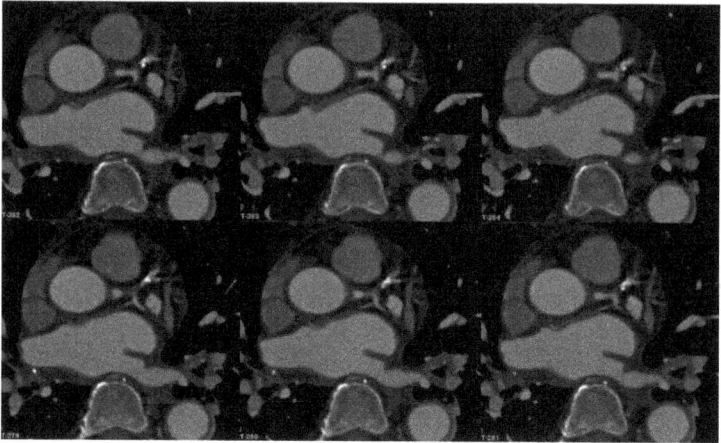

(A)

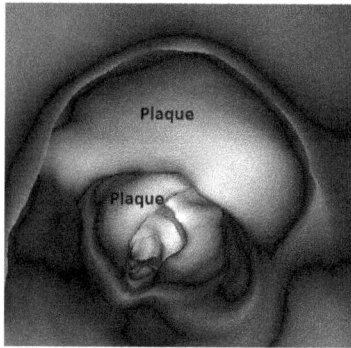

(B)

Figure 3.6. (A) 2D axial CT images show calcified plaques at the LAD artery. (B) Corresponding VIE shows calcified plaques with intraluminal protrusion resulting in significant lumen stenosis.

Non-calcified plaque is defined as any discernible structure in the coronary wall with CT attenuation lower than the contrast-enhanced lumen but higher than the surrounding tissue or pericardial fat in at least two independent planes (Fig. 3.9).[22,24,25] Recently, more detailed analysis of non-calcified plaque is proposed by some researchers to improve detection of complex composition of advanced plaques.[23,26,27] Motoyama

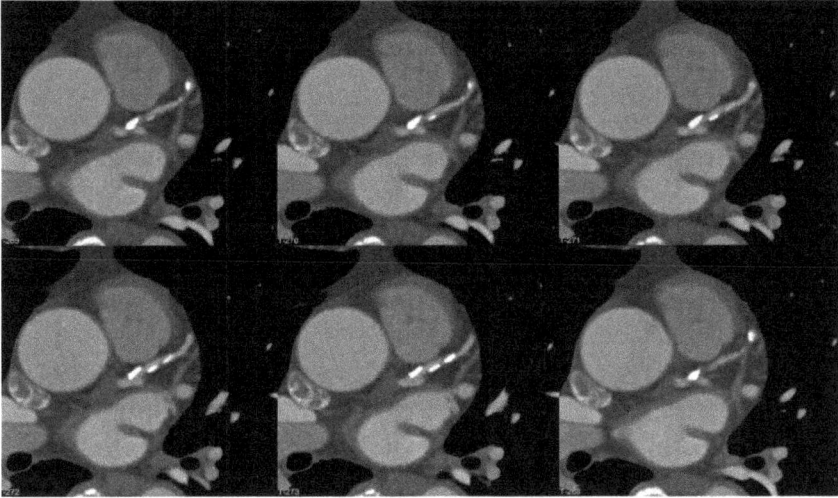

Figure 3.7. 2D axial CT images demonstrate multiple calcified plaques at the LAD artery with CT attenuation of more than 1,000 HU.

et al. classified non-calcified plaques into plaques with lipid core with CT attenuation of less than 30 HU and fibrous plaques with CT attenuation between 30 and 150 HU.[28] However, Marwan *et al.* showed a wide overlap between the lipid-rich and fibrous plaques (67 ± 31 vs 96 ± 40 HU).[29] Schlett *et al.* performed a study on human hearts and their results showed that using criteria of a threshold of 1.0 mm^2 or greater with absolute plaque area of less than 60 HU CT angiography has 69% sensitivity and 80% specificity for detection of lipid-rich plaque.[30]

Although IVUS or optical coherence tomography (OCT) is considered as the imaging modality to provide plaque classifications and quantification which are probably closest to histopathology,[31,32] CCTA has been shown to have a good agreement with these imaging modalities for accurate analysis of plaque features,[33–35] although further developments, in particular, improvement in spatial and contrast resolutions are needed to allow microscopic classification of plaque compositions.[36]

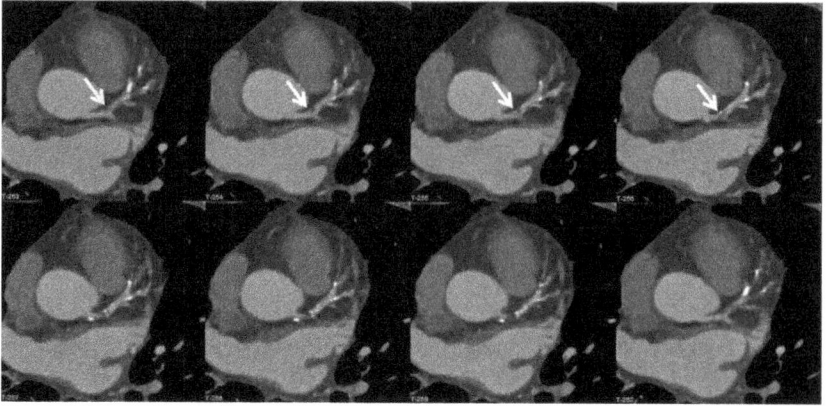

(A)

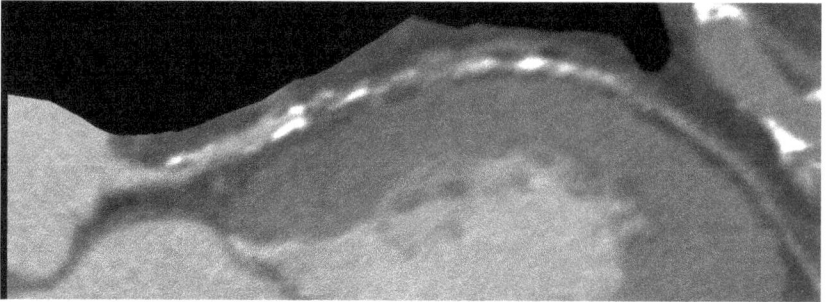

(B)

Figure 3.8. (A) 2D axial CT images show mixed plaque at the proximal segment of LAD artery. The CT attenuation of non-calcified component (arrows) is measured as 30 HU, while the calcified area is measured as 550 HU. (B) CVR image shows the mixed plaque at the proximal LAD and multiple calcified plaques at mid and distal segments of LAD.

3.4 Quantitative Assessment of Coronary Plaques

The normal coronary wall in healthy adults is about 0.15 mm (± 0.07 mm) in thickness, and this is beyond the assessment ability of spatial resolution by CCTA.[37] However, coronary plaques with clinical significance tend to be large, having a reasonable size of necrotic core ranging from 2 to 17 mm in length, and are often located in the proximal segments of coronary arteries.[9] This is within the spatial resolution limits of CCTA, thus allowing quantitative

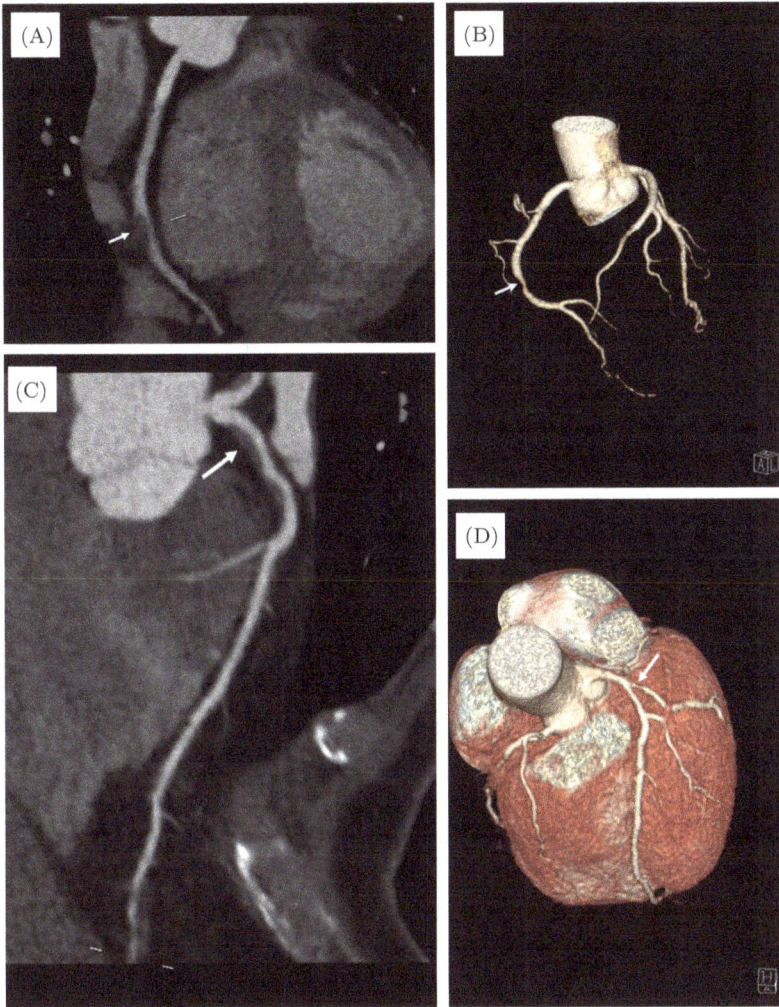

Figure 3.9. Examples of non-calcified plaques at the coronary arteries. A non-calcified plaque with significant stenosis is observed at the mid-segment of right coronary artery (arrows in A and B), and at the proximal segment of LAD coronary artery on 2D CVR and 3D VR images (arrows in C and D).

assessment of plaque features. Studies have shown that CCTA is a promising technique for plaque detection, characterization and quantification.

The most commonly used parameters for CCTA quantitative assessment of coronary plaques included plaque area and plaque volume measurements in comparison with IVUS which is considered as the reference standard. Plaque area is defined as the difference between outer vessel and lumen areas, while plaque volume is calculated as the sum of plaque areas of individual cross-sections measured on CCTA images multiplied by cross-section thickness.[22,26,38,39]

Studies based on a head to head comparison between CCTA and IVUS have concluded that CCTA has high diagnostic accuracy in the quantitative assessment of coronary plaques. Nakazato *et al.* reported a high correlation between CCTA and IVUS in the analysis of total plaque volumes with no significant differences between the two methods. Bland–Altman limits of agreement for vessel volume, lumen volume and plaque volume ranged from -53.7 to 53.1 mm^3 with a bias of -0.3 mm^3, -24.1 to 32.2 mm^3 with a bias of 4.0 mm^3, and -40.6 to 31.8 mm^3 with a bias of -4.4 mm^3, respectively.[33] Papadopoulou *et al.* presented similar findings in their study based on comparison between 64-slice CCTA and IVUS.[40] The sensitivity and specificity of CCTA for detection of coronary plaques were 86% and 71% at cross-sectional stenosis, and 96% and 88% on per segment-based analysis. Bland–Altman analysis showed a slight underestimation of any plaque volume by CCTA without reaching a significant difference. Others reported similar findings with sensitivity ranging from 95% to 97%, and specificity from 89% to 90%.[41,42]

Despite improved spatial and temporal resolution, CCTA is still inferior to IVUS for quantitative analysis of non-calcified plaques. A recent study by Sudarski *et al.* assessed dual-source CCTA in the quantitative analysis of plaque composition in 60 patients with stable CAD.[43] Their results showed that CCTA resulted in significantly lower volumes of fatty components when compared to virtual histology IVUS, while in the assessment of calcified and fibrous plaque volumes, CCTA was higher than that of IVUS. Further studies based on modern high-end CT scanners with high resolution are required to improve the diagnostic value of CCTA.

Studies based on multicenter trials also reported similar findings. The ACCURACY (assessment by coronary computed tomographic angiography of individuals undergoing invasive coronary angiography (ICA)) study is a multicenter trial consisting of 230 patients with obstructive CAD which were recruited from 16 centers and it was designed to investigate the diagnostic value of CCTA for analysis of coronary plaques in comparison with ICA.[44] On per-patient and per-segment analysis, a significant correlation was found between plaque composition and degree of coronary stenosis, with mixed plaques resulting in high rates of obstructive coronary stenosis (40.6% as confirmed by ICA), slightly less common in non-calcified plaques (27.9%), whereas calcified plaques rarely showing obstructive stenosis (0.8%) ($p = 0.02$). This further highlights the prognostic significance of using CCTA for characterization of plaque composition, consequently predicting the development of major adverse cardiac events.

CCTA also demonstrates strong correlation between adverse plaque features as assessed on CCTA and prevalence of adverse cardiac events.[45] Dey et al. in their retrospective study performed quantitative characterization of coronary plaques on CCTA in 28 patients presenting with first acute coronary syndrome (ACS) and compared with the control group with stable CAD who also underwent CCTA with ICA as the reference standard.[46] Their results showed that non-calcified plaque and low-density non-calcified plaque burdens were significantly higher in the ACS patients than the control group (57.4% vs 41.5%; 12.5% vs 8%, $p < 0.05$). On per-patient level, there was no significant difference in calcified plaque burden between ACS patients and the control group of patients. On per-vessel level, calcified plaque did not show any significant difference, however, coronary arteries with high-risk of developing ACS were found to have higher low-attenuation plaques. More details about the prognostic value of CCTA in determining major adverse cardiac events based on plaque assessment will be further discussed in Chapter 4.

Analysis of plaque composition and burden by CCTA also shows ethnic difference. In their recent study, Villadsen and colleagues compared the differences in coronary stenosis, amount and composition of coronary plaques in a cohort of Caucasian (420) and South Asian (538) patients with stable chest pain.[47] Although no significant difference was reached in total plaque burden between these two groups of patients, the Caucasian patients were found to have significantly lower non-calcified plaque composition compared to the Asian group (80.95% vs 90.42%, $p < 0.001$). Therefore, when assessing coronary plaque compositions with CCTA, ethnic factors should be taken into account.

3.5 Automatic Quantification of Coronary Plaques

One of the main limitations of CCTA lies in the fact that analysis of coronary plaque features is most commonly performed by a visual assessment, which is observer dependent, thus requiring sufficient knowledge in cardiac CT image interpretation. Furthermore, CCTA plaque quantification involves processes of manual tracing of vessel contours, image post-processing of separating epicardial fat from the coronary wall and calcified and non-calcified components, which is not only time-consuming but also introduces intra-observer variability.[48,49] Semi- or automatic quantification of coronary plaque characteristics is preferable to manual processing for improvement of the diagnostic accuracy, increase reproducibility and time-efficiency of CCTA. This has been proved in several recently published studies.

Klass *et al.* used semiautomatic plaque analysis approach for lesion segmentation and characterization, as well as quantitative analysis of plaque volumes.[50] Their results showed that larger inter-observer bias and variability existed for calcified and mixed plaques, while the lowest degree of variability was noted in non-calcified plaques. Of all types of plaques, non-calcified, mixed and calcified, the inter-observer bias and variability were 1.2%, 0.5%, 1.5%, 1.3%, and 3.3%, 4.5%, 7.0% and 4.4%, respectively, indicating the potential role of CCTA in quantitative assessment of non-calcified plaques. Dey *et al.* tested their developed automated algorithm (APQ) in 24 patients with 29 plaques as assessed on dual-source CCTA.[51] A strong correlation was found between the two observers for manual quantification of calcified and non-calcified plaque volumes (Fig. 3.10). Furthermore, the APQ showed significantly lower difference and lower bias for calcified and non-calcified plaque analysis, with excellent correlation between the observers. The same research group applied the APQ to 22 non-calcified plaques in 20 patients with correlation of CCTA findings with IVUS.[52] Excellent correlation was found between automatic quantification of plaque volume by CCTA and IVUS with corresponding mean non-calcified plaque volume being 116.6 ± 80.1 mm^3 and 105.9 ± 83.5 mm^3 for APQ and IVUS, respectively, without showing significant difference. Also, there is no significant difference in the mean absolute difference in non-calcified plaque volume between APQ and manual quantitative analysis by CT (21.2 ± 20.0 mm^3 vs

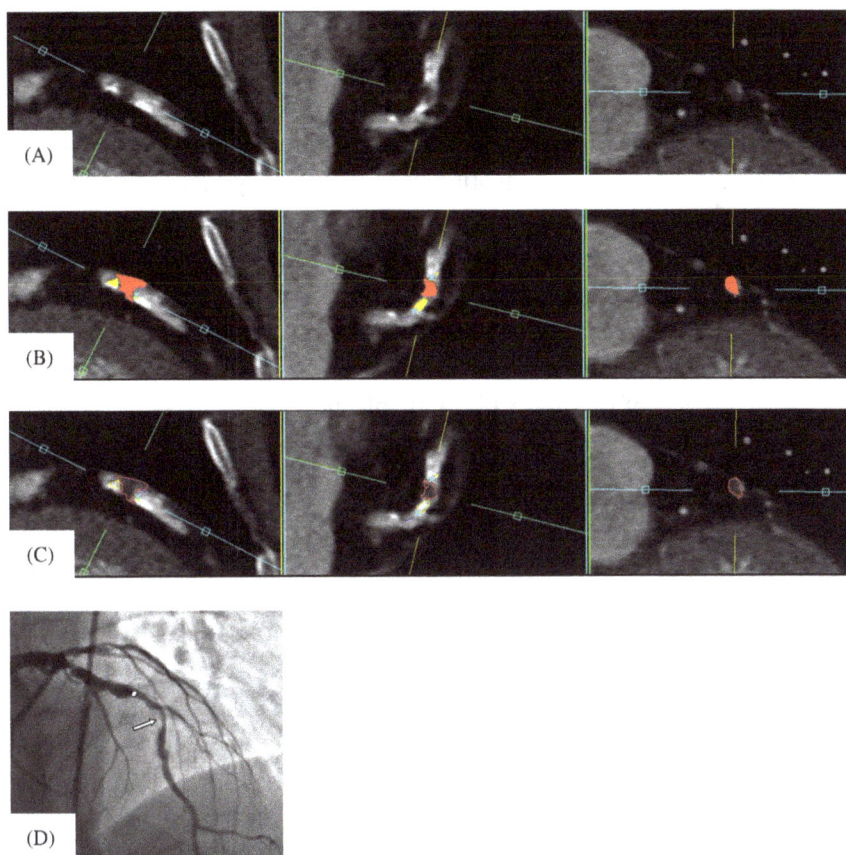

Figure 3.10. Results of automatic computer software (APQ) for plaque quantification at LAD coronary artery in a 51-year-old male patient with smoking history who was referred for CCTA. (A) MPR views showing a curved mixed plaque from the mid-LAD coronary artery. (B) Corresponding color-coded overlay from APQ quantification, with yellow overlay corresponding to calcified plaque and red overlay corresponding to non-calcified plaque. (C) APQ overlay can also be visualized as non-calcified plaque (red) and calcified plaque (yellow) contours. For this lesion, APQ calculated results were non-calcified plaque volume and calcified plaque volume 75.8 mm^3 and 14.4 mm^3, respectively, with 88% stenosis. Mean (±SD) value within the non-calcified plaque component was 81.4 ± 58.3 HU. (D) ICA confirms the mid-LAD lesion with 67% stenosis. Reprinted with permission from Dey et al.[51]

30.5 ± 30.8 mm^3). The time for automated plaque segmentation and quantification was less than 20 s, according to this study. Thus, CCTA allows for rapid and accurate quantitative measurement of non-calcified plaques compared with IVUS.

The limitation of commonly used CT-number-based plaque characterization and quantification is overcome with a novel "labeling method" proposed by Fujimoto *et al.*[53] Authors used this method to identify areas of low attenuation by comparing HU measurements in relation to adjacent areas, while differentiating low attenuation areas from image noise. They tested this novel method in 33 patients with 37 high-risk, non-calcified plaques with results compared to VH-IVUS. An excellent correlation was found between the labeling method and VH-IVUS when compared to the CT-number-based technique to measure necrotic core area. Superior correlation between the labeling method and VH-IVUS was also demonstrated for measurements of fibrous or fibrofatty plaque areas, with limits of agreement by Bland–Altman analysis for labeling method-derived measures of necrotic core area smaller than those derived by CT-number-based method $(0.3 \pm 1.1$ vs 1.8 ± 2.8 mm^2 and -2.0 to 2.5 vs -3.7 to 7.3 mm^2, respectively) (Fig. 3.11).

Automatic quantification of coronary plaques can be further enhanced by registering CCTA images with IVUS for improvement of diagnostic value. A study by Boogers *et al.* used a novel 3D registration algorithm in 50 patients comprising 146 lesions to register CCTA data with IVUS.[54] This novel approach enables registration of cardiac imaging techniques based on a slice-by-slice comparison, thus enhancing detection and quantification of coronary plaques on CCTA. Significant correlations were demonstrated between quantitative CCTA and IVUS for assessment of lumen area stenosis, plaque burden, mean plaque burden and remodeling index. Quantitative CT was shown to be reproducible for quantitative analysis of coronary plaque characteristics.

3.6 Summary

CCTA is currently a routine imaging modality for diagnostic evaluation of CAD. A number of 2D and 3D reconstructions have enhanced the diagnostic value of CCTA in the quantitative assessment of coronary plaques with accuracy comparable to the gold standard techniques, ICA and IVUS. Development of novel image post-processing tools or algorithms such as automatic quantification of coronary plaques has further augmented the clinical value of CCTA in coronary plaque analysis. The

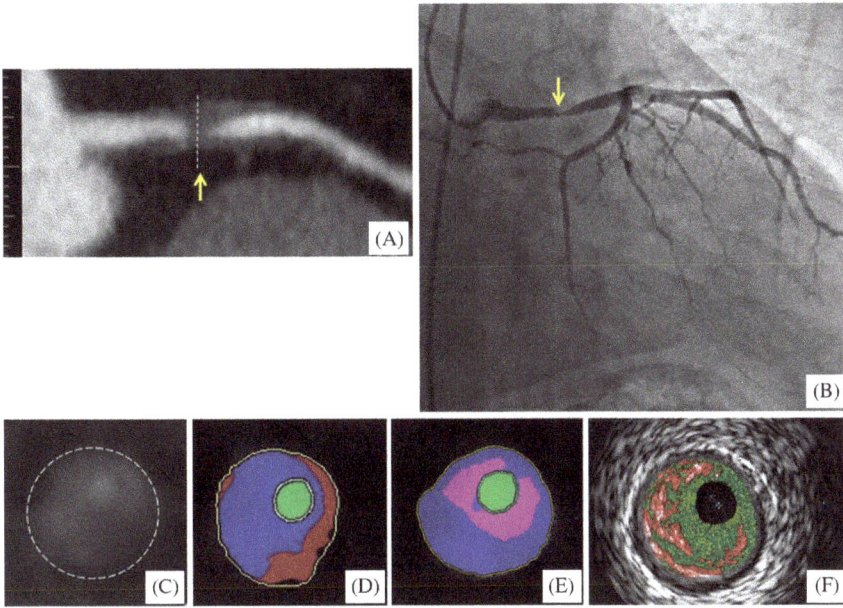

Figure 3.11. 61-year-old male who underwent CCTA and ICA with VH-IVUS. (A) and (B) Curved MPR and ICA confirm >75 % stenosis (arrow). (C) Coronary CT angiographic image orthogonal to the long axis of the left main coronary artery where the lumen diameter was minimal and plaque analysis was performed. (D) CT-number-based measurement: vessel area of 17.7 mm^2, lumen area (green) of 2.16 mm^2, necrotic core area (red) of 3.9 mm^2, and fibrous area (blue) of 11.7 mm^2. (E) Labeling method analyses: vessel area of 17.7 mm^2, lumen area (green) of 2.16 mm^2, necrotic core area (purple) of 3.8 mm^2, and fibrous area (blue) of 12.0 mm^2. (F) VH-IVUS calculated the vessel area of 18.1 mm^2, lumen area of 2.1 mm^2, necrotic core area (red) of 4.4 mm^2, and fibrous area (light green + dark green) of 8.1 mm^2. VH-IVUS virtual histology IVUS. Reprinted with permission from Fujimoto *et al.*[53]

main limitations of current studies include small sample size including small number of plaques that are analyzed in these studies, and lack of correlation CCTA findings with clinical outcomes such as development of major adverse cardiac events in patients with high-risk plaques. Further research needs to address these areas by implementing the novel quantification methods in large cohort of patients. Since CT scanners have undergone rapid developments in the last few years, high-resolution CT techniques are becoming available with significant improvements in both spatial and temporal resolution. Therefore, further studies with use of these latest CT models are necessary to provide more evidence about the improved diagnostic value of CCTA in both plaque analysis and quantification for guiding effective patient management.

References

1. Szilveszter B, Celeng C, Maurovich-Horvat P. (2016) Plaque assessment by coronary CT. *Int J Cardiovasc Imaging* **32**: 161–172.
2. Voros S. (2009) What are the potential advantages and disadvantages of volumetric CT scanning? *J Cardiovasc Comput Tomogr* **3**: 67–70.
3. Miller JM, Rochitte CE, Dewey M *et al.* (2008) Diagnostic performance of coronary angiography by 64-row CT. *N Engl J Med* **359**: 2324–2336.
4. Puchner SB, Ferencik M, Maurovich-Horvat P *et al.* (2015) Iterative image reconstruction algorithms in coronary CT angiography improve the detection of lipid-core plaque — a comparison with histology. *Eur Radiol* **25**: 15–23.
5. Oda S, Weissman G, Vembar M, Weigold WG. (2014) Iterative model reconstruction: improved image quality of low-tubevoltage prospective ECG-gated coronary CT angiography images at 256-slice CT. *Eur J Radiol* **83**: 1408–1415.
6. Takx RA, Willemink MJ, Nathoe HM *et al.* (2014) The effect of iterative reconstruction on quantitative computed tomography assessment of coronary plaque composition. *Int J Cardiovasc Imaging* **30**: 155–163.
7. Burke AP, Farb A, Malcolm GT, Lang YH, Smialek J, Virmani R. (1997) Coronary risk factors and plaque morphology in men with coronary disease who died suddenly. *N Engl J Med* **336**: 1276–1282.
8. Davies MJ. (1997) The composition of coronary artery plaques. *N Engl J Med* **336**: 1312–1314.
9. Virmani R, Burke AP, Farb A, Kolodgie FD. (2006) Pathology of the vulnerable plaque. *J Am Coll Cardiol* **47**(8 Suppl): C13–C18.
10. Naganuma T, Latib A, Costopoulos CT et al. (2014) The role of intravascular ultrasound and quantitative angiography in the functional assessment of intermediate coronary lesions: correlation with fractional flow reserve. *Cardiovasc Revasc Med* **15**(1): 3–7.
11. Jasti V, Ivan E, Yalamanchili V, Wongpraparut N, Leesar MA. (2004) Correlations between fractional flow reserve and intravascular ultrasound in patients with an ambiguous left main coronary artery stenosis. *Circulation* **110**: 2831–2836.
12. Nishioka T, Amanullah AM, Luo H *et al.* (1999) Clinical validation of intravascular ultrasound imaging for assessment of coronary stenosis severity: comparison with stress myocardial perfusion imaging. *J Am Coll Cardiol* **33**: 1870–1878.
13. Chang AM, Le J, Matsuura AC, Litt HI, Hollander JE. (2011) Does coronary artery calcium scoring add to the predictive value of coronary computed tomography angiography for adverse cardiovascular events in low-risk chest pain patients? *Acad Emerg Med* **18**: 1065–1071.

14. Kondos GT, Hoff JA, Sevrukov A *et al.* (2003) Electron-beam tomography coronary artery calcium and cardiac events: a 37-month follow-up of 5635 initially asymptomatic low- to intermediate risk adults. *Circulation* **107**: 2571–2576.

15. Eid M, De Cecco CN, Nance JW Jr *et al.* (2017) Cinematic rendering in CT: a novel, lifelike 3D visualization technique. *AJR Am J Roentgenol* **209**: 370–379.

16. Johnson PT, Schneider R, Lugo-Fagundo C, Johnson MB, Fishman EK. (2017) MDCT angiography with 3D rendering: a novel cinematic rendering algorithm for enhanced anatomic detail. *AJR Am J Roentgenol* **209**: 309–312.

17. Sun Z, Al Dosari S, Ng C, al-Muntashari A, Almaliky S. (2010) Multislice CT virtual intravascular endoscopy for assessing pulmonary embolisms: a pictorial essay. *Korean J Radiol* **11**: 222–230.

18. Sun Z, Winder J, Kelly B, Ellis P, Hirst D. (2003) CT virtual intravascular endoscopy of abdominal aortic aneurysms treated with suprarenal endovascular stent grafting. *Abdom Imaging* **28**: 580–587.

19. Sun Z, Winder RJ, Kelly BE, Ellis PK, Kennedy PT, Hirst DG. (2004) Diagnostic value of CT virtual intravascular endoscopy in aortic stent grafting. *J Endovasc Ther* **11**: 13–25.

20. Sun Z. (2013) Coronary CT angiography in coronary artery disease: correlation between virtual intravascular endoscopic appearances and left bifurcation angulation and coronary plaques. *Biomed Res Int* **2013**: 732059.

21. Schroeder S, Kopp AF, Baumbach A *et al.* (2001) Noninvasive detection and evaluation of atherosclerotic coronary plaques with multislice computed tomography. *J Am Coll Cardiol* **37**: 1430–1435.

22. Achenbach S, Moselewski F, Ropers D *et al.* (2004) Detection of calcified and non-calcified coronary atherosclerotic plaque by contrast-enhanced, submillimeter multidetector spiral computed tomography: a segment-based comparison with intravascular ultrasound. *Circulation* **109**: 14–17.

23. Hoffmann U, Moselewski F, Nieman K *et al.* (2006) Noninvasive assessment of plaque morphology and composition in culprit and stable lesions in acute coronary syndrome and stable lesions in stable angina by multidetector computed tomography. *J Am Coll Cardiol* **47**: 1655–1662.

24. Leber AW, Knez A, von Ziegler F *et al.* (2005) Quantification of obstructive and nonobstructive coronary lesions by 64-slice computed tomography: a comparative study with quantitative coronary angiography and intravascular ultrasound. *J Am Coll Cardiol* **46**: 147–154.

25. Leber AW, Knez A, Becker A *et al.* (2004) Accuracy of multidetector spiral computed tomography in identifying and differentiating the composition of coronary atherosclerotic plaques: a comparative study with intracoronary ultrasound. *J Am Coll Cardiol* **43**: 1241–1247.

26. Leber AW, Becker A, Knez A *et al.* (2006) Accuracy of 64-slice computed tomography to classify and quantify plaque volumes in the proximal coronary system: a comparative study using intravascular ultrasound. *J Am Coll Cardiol* **47**: 672–677.

27. Gao D, Ning N, Guo Y, Ning W, Niu X, Yang J. (2011) Computed tomography for detecting coronary artery plaques: a meta-analysis. *Atherosclerosis* **219**: 603–609.
28. Motoyama S, Kondo T, Sarai M *et al.* (2007) Multislice computed tomographic characteristics of coronary lesions in acute coronary syndromes. *J Am Coll Cardiol* **50**: 319–326.
29. Marwan M, Taher MA, El Meniawy K *et al.* (2011) In vivo CT detection of lipid-rich coronary artery atherosclerotic plaques using quantitative histogram analysis: a head to head comparison with IVUS. *Atherosclerosis* **215**: 110–115.
30. Schlett CL, Maurovich-Horvat P, Ferencik M *et al.* (2013) Histogram analysis of lipid-core plaques in coronary computed tomographic angiography: ex vivo validation against histology. *Invest Radiol* **48**: 646–653.
31. Briguori C, Anzuini A, Airoldi F *et al.* (2001) Intravascular ultrasound criteria for the assessment of the functional significance of intermediate coronary artery stenoses and comparison with fractional flow reserve. *Am J Cardiol* **87**: 136–141.
32. Leschka S, Seitun S, Dettmer M *et al.* (2010) Ex vivo evaluation of coronary atherosclerotic plaques: characterization with dual-source CT in comparison with histopathology. *J Cardiovasc Comput Tomogr* **4**: 301–308.
33. Nakazato R, Shalev A, Doh JH *et al.* (2013) Quantification and characterisation of coronary artery plaque volume and adverse plaque features by coronary computed tomographic angiography: a direct comparison to intravascular ultrasound. *Eur Radiol* **23**: 2109–2117.
34. Pundziute G, Schuijf JD, Jukema JW *et al.* (2008) Head-to-head comparison of coronary plaque evaluation between multislice computed tomography and intravascular ultrasound radiofrequency data analysis. *JACC Cardiovasc Interv* **1**: 176–182.
35. Voros S, Rinehart S, Qian Z *et al.* (2011) Prospective validation of standardized, 3-dimensional, quantitative coronary computed tomographic plaque measurements using radiofrequency backscatter intravascular ultrasound as reference standard in intermediate coronary arterial lesions: results from the ATLANTA (Assessment of Tissue Characteristics, Lesion Morphology, and Hemodynamics by Angiography with Fractional Flow Reserve, Intravascular Ultrasound and Virtual Histology, and Noninvasive Computed Tomography in Atherosclerotic Plaques) I Study. *JACC Cardiovasc Imaging* **4**: 198–205.
36. Sarem F, Achenbach S. (2015) Coronary plaque characterization using CT. *AJR Am J Roentgen* **204**: W249–W260.
37. Nissen SE, Yock P. (2001) Intravascular ultrasound: novel pathophysiological insights and current clinical applications. *Circulation* **103**: 604–616.
38. Moselewski F, Ropers D, Pohle K *et al.* (2004) Comparison of measurement of cross-sectional coronary atherosclerotic plaque and vessel areas by 16-slice multidetector computed tomography versus intravascular ultrasound. *Am J Cardiol* **94**: 1294–1297.

39. Achenbach S, Ropers D, Hoffmann U *et al.* (2004) Assessment of coronary remodeling in stenotic and nonstenotic coronary atherosclerotic lesions by multidetector spiral computed tomography. *J Am Coll Cardiol* **43**: 842–847.

40. Papadopoulou SL, Neefjes LA, Schaap M *et al.* (2011) Detection and quantification of coronary atherosclerotic plaque by 64-slice multidetector CT: a systematic head-to-head comparison with intravascular ultrasound. *Atherosclerosis* **219**: 163–170.

41. Sun J, Zhang Z, Lu B *et al.* (2008) Identification and quantification of coronary atherosclerotic plaques: a comparison of 64-MDCT and intravascular ultrasound. *AJR Am J Roentgenol* **190**: 748–754.

42. Petranovic M, Soni A, Bezzera H *et al.* (2009) Assessment of nonstenotic coronary lesions by 64-slice multidetector computed tomography in comparison to intravascular ultrasound: evaluation of nonculprit coronary lesions. *J Cardiovasc Comput Tomogr* **3**: 24–31.

43. Sudarski S, Fink C, Sueseibeck T *et al.* (2013) Quantitative analysis of coronary plaque morphology by dual-source CT in patients with acute non-ST elevation myocardial infarction compared to patients with stable coronary artery disease correlated with virtual histology intravascular ultrasound. *Acad Radiol* **20**: 995–1003.

44. Min JK, Edwardes M, Lin FY *et al.* (2011) Relationship of coronary artery plaque composition to coronary artery stenosis severity: results from the prospective multicenter ACCURACY trial. *Atherosclerosis* **219**: 573–578.

45. Dey D, Schuhbaeck A, Min JK, Berman DS, Achenbach S. (2013) Non-invasive measurement of coronary plaque from coronary CT angiography and its clinical implications. *Expert Rev Cardiovasc Ther* **11**: 1067–1077.

46. Dey D, Achenbach S, Schuhbaeck A *et al.* (2014) Comparison of quantitative atherosclerotic plaque burden from coronary CT angiography in patients with first acute coronary syndrome and stable coronary artery disease. *J Cardiovasc Comput Tomogr* **8**: 368–374.

47. Villadsen PR, Petersen SE, Dey D *et al.* (2017) Coronary atherosclerotic plaque burden and composition by CT angiography in Caucasian and South Asian patients with stable chest pain. *Eur Heart J Cardiovasc Imaging.* **18**(5): 556–567.

48. Burgstahler C, Reimann A, Beck T *et al.* (2007) Influence of a lipid-lowering therapy on calcified and noncalcified coronary plaques monitored by multislice detector computed tomography: results of the New Age II Pilot Study. *Invest Radiol* **42**: 189–195.

49. Schmid M, Achenbach S, Ropers D *et al.* (2008) Assessment of changes in non-calcified atherosclerotic plaque volume in the left main and left anterior descending coronary arteries over time by 64-slice computed tomography *Am J Cardiol* **101**: 579–584.

50. Klass O, Kleihans S, Walker MJ *et al.* (2010) Coronary plaque imaging with 256-slice multidetector computed tomography: interobserver variability of volumetric lesion parameters with semiautomatic plaque analysis software. *Int J Cardiovasc Imaging* **26**: 711–720.

51. Dey D, Cheng VY, Slomka PJ *et al.* (2009) Automated 3-dimensional quantification of noncalcified and calcified coronary plaque from coronary CT angiography. *J Cardiovasc Comput Tomogr* **3**: 372–382.
52. Dey D, Schepis T, Marwan M *et al.* (2010) Automated three-dimensional quantification of noncalcified coronary plaque from coronary CT angiography: comparison with intravascular US. *Radiology* **257**: 516–522.
53. Fujimoto S, Kondo T, Kodama T *et al.* (2014) A novel method for non-invasive plaque morphology analysis by coronary computed tomography angiography. *Int J Cardiovasc Imaging* **30**: 1373–1382.
54. Boogers MJ, Broersen A, van Velzen JE *et al.* (2012) Automated quantification of coronary plaque with computed tomography: comparison with intravascular ultrasound using a dedicated registration algorithm for fusion-based quantification. *Eur Heart J* **33**: 1007–1016.

4 Coronary CT Angiography: Quantitative Assessment of Coronary Plaques

Table of Contents

Abstract

In Chapter 3, coronary computed tomography angiography (CCTA) characterization and assessment of coronary plaques was discussed, but with a focus on 2D and 3D visualizations of plaques. This chapter mainly deals with the quantitative analysis of plaque features or components by CCTA with corresponding clinical significance in the diagnostic assessment of coronary artery disease (CAD). Identification of specific morphological plaque features on CCTA is of paramount importance to diagnose high-risk patients and guide effective patient management. The purpose of this chapter is to discuss the clinical value of CCTA in the diagnostic assessment of plaques with the aim of identifying vulnerable plaques, therefore, achieving the goal of predicting and preventing major adverse cardiac events.

Keywords: coronary computed tomography angiography, coronary plaque, diagnosis, detection, feature, quantitative assessment.

4.1 Introduction

Coronary computed tomography angiography (CCTA) has become a standard diagnostic tool for patients with suspected coronary artery disease (CAD) in many clinical centers with high diagnostic value reported in the literature.[1–5] Cardiac CT imaging has undergone rapid technological developments over the last decade which has led to the improvement of diagnostic spectrum of CCTA in the quantitative analysis of coronary plaques, in addition to the conventional assessment of coronary lumen stenosis. These include characterization of plaque composition in relation to the corresponding clinical outcomes such as prediction of major adverse cardiac events.[6–9]

Identification of plaque components, in particular, differentiation of vulnerable plaques from stable ones is more significant than detection of lumen stenosis because there is a close association between plaque composition and myocardial ischemia and development of adverse cardiac events.[10–13] Therefore, the current trend of CCTA in the diagnosis of CAD has shifted from previous coronary lumen assessment of degree of stenosis to quantitative analysis of plaque features because the degree of lumen stenosis does not always translate to myocardial ischemic changes.[14] This chapter provides a comprehensive review of CCTA in the visualization and characterization of coronary plaque characteristics, specifically focusing on plaque composition analysis for identification of high-risk plaques.

4.2 Overview of Diagnostic Value of CCTA

Since its introduction in 2004, 64-slice CT scanners are considered prerequisite for CCTA in routine clinical practice.[6] According to several systematic reviews and meta-analyses, the sensitivities and specificities of CCTA are generally more than 97% and 87% in most of the studies using 64-slice CT in the diagnosis of CAD.[15–20] These analyses prove that CCTA has high diagnostic value in the detection and characterization of coronary artery stenosis.

Currently, 320-slice or second generation of 320-slice or third generation of dual-source CT represents the latest technological developments in coronary CT imaging with improved diagnostic performance. Advancements of multislice CT systems from a 64-slice to 640-slice system allow accurate assessment of stenosis severity and atherosclerotic plaque composition, or feasibility of the acquisition of whole-heart coverage within a single heart beat in one gantry rotation. There are three systematic reviews and meta-analyses of 320-slice CCTA available in the literature, and these analyses have further confirmed the high diagnostic accuracy of 320-slice CCTA in CAD.[21–23] The mean diagnostic sensitivity is similar to that reported in the 64-slice CCTA, but the mean specificity of 320-slice CCTA is higher than that of 64-slice CCTA studies, showing the improved diagnostic value of 320-slice CCTA for excluding coronary artery stenosis. However, we need to be aware of the fact that diagnostic performance of 320-slice CCTA is similar to that of 64- and 128-slice for the detection of ≥50% coronary artery stenosis because its temporal resolution is still inferior to that of 64-slice or 128-slice CT, despite the extended z-axis coverage of 320-slice CT when compared to 64- or 128-slice CT scanners.[24] Table 4.1 is a summary of the systematic reviews/meta-analyses of diagnostic value of CCTA comparing 320-slice CT with 64-slice CT.

The second generation of 320-slice CT shows improved diagnostic value when compared to the first generation of 320-slice or 64-/256-slice CT. The temporal resolution has been improved from 175 ms to 137 ms due to faster gantry rotation, and excellent image quality has been achieved with use of iterative reconstruction with resultant low radiation dose.[25–27] Ghekiere et al. in their prospective study reported the diagnostic value of second-generation 320-slice CCTA in 200 consecutive patients with median calcium score of 63. Their results showed that the low rate of non-diagnostic segments due to motion-related artifacts is 0.2%, which is much lower than corresponding rates of 1.9%, 1.3% and

Table 4.1. Diagnostic value of CCTA in CAD according to systematic reviews and meta-analyses.

Type of CT scan	First author	No. of articles in the analysis	Patient-based sensitivity (95% CI)	Patient-based specificity (95% CI)
64-slice CCTA	Abdulla et al.[16]	27 studies	97.5% (96–99)	91% (87.5–94)
	Stein et al.[17]	23 studies	98% (96–98)	88% (85–89)
	Mowatt et al.[18]	28 studies	99% (97–99)	89% (83–94)
	Sun et al.[15]	15 studies	97% (94–99)	88% (79–97)
	Guo et al.[19]	24 studies	98% (99–99)	87% (83–90)
	Salavati et al.[20]	25 studies	99% (97–99)	89% (84–92)
320-slice CCTA	Gaudio et al.[21]	7 studies	95.4% (88.8–98.2)	94.7% (89.1–97.5)
	Li et al.[22]	10 studies	93% (91–95)	86% (82–89)
	Sun and Lin[23]	12 studies	96.3% (92.9–99.8)	86.4% (77.8–94.9)

Note: CCTA — coronary CT angiography.

3% using 64-, 256-slice and high-pitch dual-source CCTA, respectively.[28–30] Image quality was mainly affected by the coronary calcifications but less influenced by patient's heart rate or body mass index (BMI).[27]

Over the last few years, the third-generation dual-source CT was introduced to allow acquisition of 192 slices per rotation with wider detector coverage. Further improvement in gantry rotation time to 250 ms results in a temporal resolution of 66 ms, which is superior to the 75 ms from the previous second-generation dual-source CT, and much better than that from 320-slice CT.[31–33] High diagnostic value can be achieved with improved scan speed and other technical advances such as advanced iterative reconstructions and automatic tube voltage selection, regardless of the BMI. Mangold et al. compared the diagnostic value of CCTA in 76 patients with non-obese (BMI) <30 kg/m^2 and obese (>30 kg/m^2) using third-generation dual-source CT.[34] No significant differences were found in sensitivity, specificity, positive predictive value and negative predictive value between obese and non-obese patients on per-patient, per-vessel and per-segment analysis ($p > 0.05$). In addition, the volume of contrast medium was reduced with mean volume of 71 and 77 mL for non-obese and obese patients, respectively. With use of automatic tube voltage section, the effective dose was 3.3 mSv for the protocol of tube voltage <120 kV as opposed to the 10.2 mSv for 120 kV protocol.[34] Further dose reduction can be achieved with use of high-pitch CCTA protocols or a combination with iterative reconstruction algorithms and low tube voltages.

A recent study has demonstrated the mean effective dose of 1.3 mSv in 186 patients who underwent propsectively ECG-triggered high-pitch CCTA.[35] Of all coronary artery segments, 98.5% were rated as diagnostic, with sensitivity, specificity, positive predictive value, negative predictive value and diagnostic accuracy being 90.1%, 97.4%, 82%, 98.6%, and 96.5% on a per-vessel assessment.[35] Currently, the low-dose CCTA protocols are available in clinical practice, with dose values significantly reduced to even lower than that of invasive coronary angiography (ICA). Effective dose reduction to less than 1 mSv is achievable with the modern CT scanners, and ultra-low-dose CCTA has been also reported in some recent studies with the mean radiation dose of less than 0.4 mSv. This indicates that the effective dose of CCTA is comparable to a 2-view chest X-ray examination.[36–40] These studies further confirm that CCTA with the use of latest dose-reduction strategies has become a reality to serve as an effective alternative to ICA with low radiation dose, but in the meantime maintaining diagnostic image quality.

4.3 Quantitative Assessment of Coronary Plaques

Traditionally, it is believed that acute coronary syndrome (ACS) is caused by coronary lesions with severe stenosis (>70%).[41] However, most of the cardiac events are found to result from angiographically mild stenosis (<50%), according to the PROSPECT trial.[42] Plaque rupture represents the most common presentation which accounts for two-thirds of all cardiac events, while plaque erosion with development of thrombus is responsible for about one-third cases, and less than 5% of cardiac events are related to calcified nodules/lesions or other causes.[43–45]

Great effort has been made in plaque imaging and the focus is placed to identify factors that trigger the ACS, or identify patients at high risk of developing ACS. This leads to the paradigm shift of CCTA in coronary plaque imaging with the research direction changed from the previously focused detection of coronary luminal narrowing to the currently concentrated characterization of plaque morphological features. This strategy is based on the fact that recent evidence shows the capability of CCTA to look beyond the coronary lumen and quantitative assessment of plaque features assists development of personalized medicine to therapeutic interventions for prevention and reduction of cardiac events.[46]

Intravascular ultrasound (IVUS) and optical coherence tomography (OCT) allow quantitative plaque characterization, however, both are invasive imaging modalities, thus they are not widely available in clinical practice. As a less invasive modality with widespread applications, CCTA is able to provide detailed analysis of plaque morphology and components which add incremental prognostic value in CAD. Nadjiri and colleagues in their study, published in 2016, for the first time reported the predictive value of plaque analysis by CCTA. Authors performed comprehensive analysis of plaque features including low-attenuation plaque volume, positive remodeling index, napkin-ring sign and spotty calcification in 1,168 patients with suspected CAD. The mean follow-up was 5.7 years.[47] Although all plaque features were associated with major adverse cardiac events, low-attention plaque volume was found to demonstrate the strongest association, indicating an independent predictor of cardiac events ($p < 0.0001$). It provides additional prognostic value beyond other factors to improve risk prediction.[47]

The following sections will focus on the quantitative analysis of these plaque features by CCTA. As discussed above, there are mainly four plaque characteristics which determine the plaque vulnerability, namely: low-attenuation area, positive remodeling index, napkin-ring sign and spotty calcification. Calcified plaques are already well known in the diagnostic assessment of CAD, and they represent stable atherosclerotic situation, while these four plaque features play an important role in the identification of vulnerability or risk factors responsible for plaque to rupture. Therefore, accurate assessment of these components contributes to the clinical detection of vulnerable plaques.

4.3.1 Low-Attenuation Area

The clinical importance of using CT for analysis of plaque components is to detect vulnerable plaque at the individual patient level, therefore, identifying those individuals at potential risk of developing myocardial infarction or other adverse cardiac events. Most ischemic cardiac events are provoked by rupture of a plaque which is rich in lipid, inflammatory and necrotic material, and covered by a thin fibrous cap.[48] Thus, differentiation of lipid-rich plaques from fibrous plaques represents the focus of current studies with the aim of providing valuable information about plaque vulnerability (Fig. 4.1).[49]

An early study reported the feasibility of using CCTA to demonstrate plaque attenuation based on CT attenuation measurements, with soft plaques having lower CT numbers than intermediate and calcified plaques.[50] Later reports have further confirmed the differences between

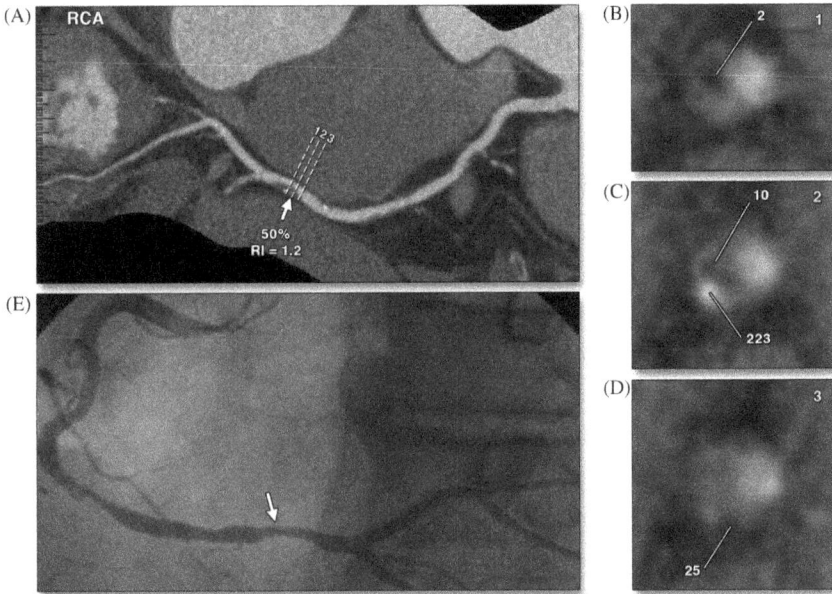

Figure 4.1. Low-attenuation high-risk plaque in a 66-year-old male with atypical chest pain. (A) Curved planar reformatted CT image shows 50% stenosis at the distal segment of right coronary artery (RCA). (B)–(D) Cross-sectional analysis reveals high-risk plaque features: a low-attenuation plaque area adjacent to the lumen (2–25 HU), spotty calcification (223 HHU), and positive remodeling (remodeling index 1.2). (E) ICA confirms the lumen stenosis <50%. Reprinted with permission under the open access from Hecht *et al.*[49]

different types of plaques according to plaque components: calcified, non-calcified and mixed plaques. Significant difference was found in CT attenuation in terms of Hounsfield units (HUs) between calcified and non-calcified plaques.[51-53] An *ex vivo* study comparing IVUS and CCTA showed the mean CT attenuation of 47 ± 9 HU for lipid-rich plaques, and 104 ± 28 HU for predominantly fibrotic plaques.[54] Similar findings were reported by another study which used histogram analysis of the intraplaque CT attenuation with lipid-rich plaques having lower mean CT numbers (76 ± 31 HU) when compared to the mean CT numbers of 96 ± 40 HU for fibrotic plaques.[55]

CCTA has been shown to correlate well with IVUS in terms of plaque composition differentiation with soft plaques, soft plaques with thrombus and fibrotic plaques having 32.9 ± 8.7 HU, 43.2 ± 10.7 HU, and 82.5 ± 22.6 HU, respectively.[56] These findings indicate that vulnerable plaques associated with ACS have lower CT numbers due to its components of thin fibrotic cap and large necrotic core, while stable plaques tend to have higher CT numbers because of fibrotic or calcified lesions.[57]

A longitudinal study with a mean follow up of 27 months by Motoyama and colleagues demonstrated that low-attenuation plaques (<30 HU) were more frequently seen in patients who developed ACS compared to those with stable angina pectoris ($p < 0.01$).[58] Low-attenuation plaque volume was significantly larger in patients who developed ACS than those who did not (20.4 ± 3.4 mm^3 vs 1.1 ± 1.4 mm^3, $p < 0.001$). Results from the ATLANTA study reported similar findings. This prospective single-center study involved 60 patients with intermediate coronary lesions (40–70% stenosis), with IVUS/virtual histology used as the reference method for quantitative analysis of plaque features. The mean follow-up period was 12 months. The most important findings of this study lie in two aspects: plaques with less calcified and more non-calcified components were found in coronary lesions with major adverse cardiovascular events (MACE); higher percentage of fibrofatty tissue was noticed at the minimal lumen area associated with MACE.[59]

Currently, research focus of CCTA is to conduct quantitative analysis of CT characteristics of vulnerable plaques based on the comparison so as to guide therapeutic approaches for individual patients in order to prevent and reduce cardiac events. Although it is difficult to reliably differentiate lipid-rich from fibrous lesions based on CT attenuation,[46,60] low-attenuation plaques with average CT attenuation less than 30 HU were more often seen in patients with ACS than those with stable angina pectoris (79% vs 9%, $p < 0.0001$).[57] Most of the studies used 30 HU as a cut-off value to determine low-attenuation plaque, however, its CT attenuation value could range from 30 to 60 HU according to different reports.[57,58,61–63] This may be due to several reasons. Frist, the CT attenuation of a coronary plaque could be variable depending on the degree of coronary lumen enhancement and scanning protocols (kV setting and CT system including slice thickness, reconstruction algorithms or kernels).[64,65] Second, measurement of CT density of low-attenuation plaque differs from study to study due to use of different approaches in determining the size of regions of interest.[61,66] While results from current studies are promising, more large-scale, multi-center clinical studies with long-term follow-up are warranted to verify the clinical value of CCTA in the characterization of coronary plaques.

4.3.2 Positive Remodeling Index

Although assessment of coronary lumen stenosis is the most common parameter to determine significant coronary stenosis, rupture-prone plaques might not be associated with significant lumen narrowing.[67] Positive vascular remodeling is described as a compensatory enlargement in the vessel size that occurs at the location of the coronary plaque with the increase of plaque size, the cross-sectional luminal area is preserved,[68] while decrease in vessel size is defined as negative remodeling due to vessel shrinkage.[69,70] Positive remodeling has become an increasing research topic in recent years and has been shown to be associated with the large quantity of macrophages and increased necrotic core,[71] therefore, it is considered as a reliable sign to indicate plaque vulnerability.

CCTA can measure vascular wall and coronary lumen changes, thus calculating the remodeling index which is currently used to determine if the coronary lesions have positive remodeling. The remodeling index is defined as the ratio of the cross-sectional area (or diameter) at the site of maximal stenosis to a normal reference cross-sectional area (or diameter).[72–74] A remodeling index of >1.0 is suggested for diagnosing positive remodeling as assessed by CCTA, while some studies use the index of ≥ 1.05 or ≥ 1.1.[74,75] Studies have demonstrated the association between positive remodeling and vulnerable plaques in patients who develop ACS. Studies comparing CCTA with IVUS or OCT showed that coronary plaques with positive remodeling index on CCTA have a higher plaque burden, a large amount of necrotic core and most likely a high prevalence of thin-cap fibroatheroma compared to those lesions without having positive remodeling index.[76,77] Cross-sectional studies have shown the higher remodeling index in patients with ACS than those with stable angina pectoris (Fig. 4.2) ($p < 0.05$).[78,79] In a representative study involving more than 1,000 patients with a mean follow-up of 27 months, authors reported that positive remodeling index and low-attenuation plaques were indicators to detect patients at a higher risk of developing ACS than those without these plaque features.[58]

A cut-off value of remodeling index is recommended as >1.1 as this has been shown to improve the specificity from 45% to 78%.[74] However, a more recent study used a higher threshold for remodeling index of >1.4 as suggested by previous reports indicating the possible higher remodeling index for non-stenotic plaques.[80–82] Conte *et al.* in their study enrolled 265 patients with non-obstructive coronary plaques (<50% stenosis) with a mean follow-up of 98 ± 20 months.[80] Coronary plaque characteristics including positive remodeling index (>1.4), low-attenuation plaque (<30 HU), plaque burden area, napkin-ring sign and spotty calcification were analyzed in relation to the development of major adverse cardiac events. Their results showed that positive remodeling index of >1.1 was not predictive of all cardiac events at follow-up. When the index was adjusted for >1.4, all events were associated with presence of remodeling index >1.4, low-attenuation plaques and plaque burden areas ($p < 0.05$). This study represents the longest follow-up so far in comparison with previous studies. Further, they suggested a higher cut-off value of >1.4 to predict hard cardiac events when compared with others using >1.1. The study shows promising plaque characteristics for detecting cardiac events in patients with non-obstructive CAD, although further research with a larger number of patients is required to confirm the value of plaque features as assessed on CCTA in clinical practice.

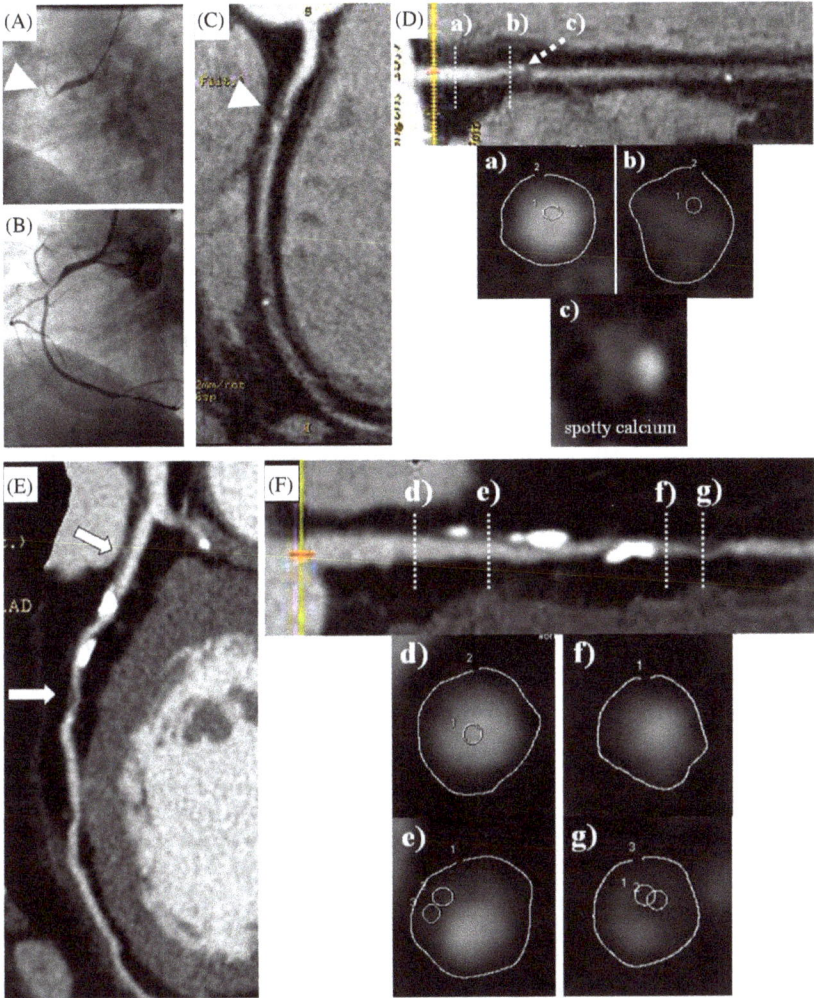

Figure 4.2.   CCTA and ICA in a 58-year-old man with non-ST-segment elevated myocardial infarction. (A) and (B) ICA shows occlusion of RCA with a recanalization of the lesion. (C) and (D) Curved planar reformation images show non-calcified plaque with spotty calcification in the proximal segment of RCA (arrowhead). The cross-sectional views show vessel areas of the reference site (a) and non-calcified plaque (b) being 23 and 29 mm^2, respectively. Thus, the remodeling index is 1.26. The minimum CT attenuation of the non-calcified plaque is 16 HU. (E) and (F) Curved planar reformatted images show multiple non-culprit non-calcified plaques in the left anterior descending coronary artery (arrows). The cross-sectional views demonstrate vessel areas of the reference site (d) and non-obstructive non-calcified plaque (e) being 28 and 28 mm^2, respectively. Thus, the remodeling index is 1.0. The minimum CT attenuation of the non-calcified plaque is −7 HU. Reprinted with permission from Kitagawa *et al.*[79]

4.3.3 Napkin Ring Sign

The napkin-ring sign is an anatomic feature visualized within the soft plaque. This sign is recently proposed as a specific CT feature associated with plaque vulnerability and development of ACS.[83–85] A ring-like enhancement of CT attenuation is used to describe this specific attenuation pattern that is seen in the non-calcified plaque.[86] This feature is different from low-attenuation plaque and positive remodeling index as it is a qualitative plaque feature which is defined by the presence of two features in a non-calcified plaque: a central low CT attenuation area which is in close contact with the coronary lumen; and a ring-like higher attenuation area surrounding this central area (Fig. 4.3).[84, 86]

Studies have shown the association between napkin-ring sign and high-risk plaques as well as prevalence of ACS. In their *ex vivo* study involving seven human donor hearts, Seifarth *et al.* analyzed histopathological features of atherosclerotic plaques observed in CCTA.[87] Authors reported that the necrotic core area was twice the size in plaques with a napkin-ring sign compared to those without this sign (1.10 mm^2 vs 0.46 mm^2, $p = 0.05$). Further, plaques with napkin-ring sign were two-fold of those without the sign (10.15 mm^2 vs 6.36 mm^2), indicating a potential

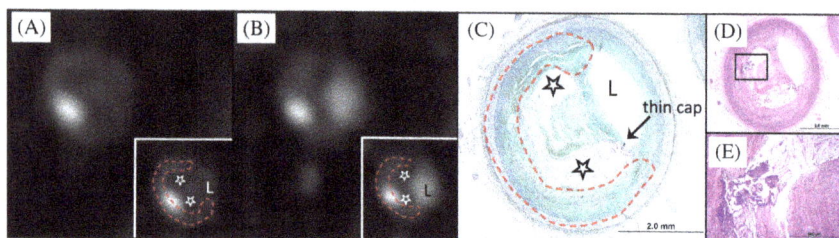

Figure 4.3. Cross-sectional views of a coronary plaque with napkin-ring sign and spotty calcification. The circumferential outer rim (red dashed line) of the non-calcified plaque is observed on non-contrast (A) and contrast-enhanced CT images (B) with low CT attenuation (44 ± 8.8 HU, range 23–61 HU, vs 48.6 ± 5.8 HU, range 34–60.5 HU, respectively) as compared to the central part of the plaque with corresponding CT attenuation of 27.9 ± 4.2 HU (range 20.7–36.4 HU) and 31 ± 6.6 HU (range 19–44 HU) on non-contrast and contrast-enhanced CT images. (C)–(E) Histological sections reveal a late fibroatheroma with spotty calcification. The lesion is characterized by a necrotic core (star), which is consistent with a significant amount of fibrous plaque tissue as seen on CT images. Arrowheads point to the *vasa vasorum* and L refers to lumen. Reprinted with permission from Maurovich-Horvat *et al.*[86]

marker of napkin-ring sign for advanced plaques.[87] A prospective study involving 895 patients with a mean follow-up of more than 12 months has further confirmed the predictive value of napkin-ring sign for developing ACS.[88] Napkin-ring sign is one of the independent predictive factors ($p < 0.0001$) for future ACS events. Kaplan–Meier analysis demonstrated the association between plaques with napkin-ring sign and a higher risk of ACS events.[88]

In a recent study with a long-term follow-up of more than 8 years, napkin-ring sign is one of the indicators associated with significantly higher cardiac events.[80] The ability of CCTA for detecting the attenuation change within coronary plaques was confirmed by a recent study. Yang *et al.* performed a direct head-to-head comparison of CCTA characteristics of plaque features with OCT-defined thin cap fibroatheroma in 28 symptomatic patients.[89] Low-attenuation plaque and napkin-ring sign as shown on CCTA were significantly correlated with OCT ($p < 0.05$), although OCT showed higher frequency of detecting these high-risk plaque indicators compared to CCTA. Results from the ROMICAT II (Rule Out Myocardial Infarction/Ischemia Using Computer-Assisted Tomography) trial further highlight the clinical value of CCTA in quantitative analysis of high-risk plaque morphology,[90] however, low-attenuation plaque, positive remodeling index and plaque burden were found to be significantly associated with high-risk plaque features.

Although clinical studies reported high specificity (96–100%) of napkin-ring sign for the identification of vulnerable coronary lesions,[66,74] as well as high specificity (98.9% and 94.1%) for identification of advanced plaques and thin-cap fibroatheroma,[84] the napkin-ring sign has a low sensitivity of 42% and positive predictive value of 22% for determining future ACS events.[88] Further research is necessary to provide a more detailed analysis of plaque features, in particular, focusing on the differentiation of plaque attenuation patterns to develop reliable plaque classification scheme so that improved diagnostic performance of CCTA in the detection of vulnerable plaques could be achieved.[46, 91]

4.3.4 Spotty Calcification

This is a direct relationship between coronary artery calcification and the extent and severity of atherosclerotic CAD.[92–94] Thus, calcification in the coronary plaques as assessed by CT-based calcium scoring is a strong indicator of predicting cardiac events. Quantifying the amount of calcification which is commonly defined as coronary calcium scoring has been widely accepted as a risk stratification schemed for patients with suspected CAD, and for screening risk of future cardiac events. This is usually quantified by using the Agatston score or the volume score or calcium mass.[95]

Clinical value of assessing degree of coronary calcification has been supported by evidence showing that the absence of calcium reliably excludes obstructive coronary artery stenosis, and that the amount of calcium in coronary arteries is a robust predictor for risk assessment of cardiovascular events. Studies have shown that a very low risk of cardiac events was observed in patients with zero or no coronary calcification (<1%), while significantly increased risk of cardiac events were found in patients with high degree of calcification or extensive coronary calcification, with an increase of up to 11-fold reported in some studies.[96–99] The prognostic value of coronary calcium scoring has been well addressed in some studies.[100–103] Some recent reports based on long-term follow-up or multicenter experience have further confirmed the clinical value of coronary calcium scoring for improvement of prediction, reclassification of individuals at risk for future cardiac events and a more accurate predictor of significant coronary stenosis than conventional risk factors.[104–106]

Despite clinical validation of association between coronary calcium and degree of atherosclerosis and prediction of cardiac events, the effect of coronary calcification on plaque vulnerability is controversial.[107–109] This is mainly because of the fact that most plaques with severe calcification are clinically quiescent, whereas only microcalcification or spotty/small calcification was found to be associated with disease progression or predictive of vulnerable plaque features (Fig. 4.3).[86,110] In their study Ehara *et al.* presented the first experience of using IVUS to demonstrate the relationship between spotty calcification and vulnerable coronary lesions and ACS. Their analysis showed that spotty calcification with a fibrofatty plaque was more frequently seen in patients with ACS and unstable angina pectoris compared with the stable angina pectoris patients ($p < 0.0005$). In contrast, the frequency of extensive calcification was the highest in patients with stable angina pectoris. Therefore, coronary plaques with extensive calcifications indicate fibrous atherosclerotic changes, while small calcium deposits are likely to be associated with plaque vulnerability along with other plaque features such as low-attenuation plaque and with positive remodeling.[110]

Spotty calcification on CCTA is defined as a small dense plaque area with CT attenuation of >130 HU and is surrounded by non-calcified plaque. Some studies proposed the cut-off value to define spotty calcification as <3 mm,[57,58] while others determined the spotty calcification based on the following criterion: a coronary lesion comprising small calcium deposits within an arc of <90°. If the coronary lesion contains moderate or extensive calcification with an arc of 90°–180° or >180°, it is defined as intermediate or severe calcification.[105] Due to different criteria used as well as some kind of uncertainty in the relationship between spotty calcification and plaque vulnerability,[111] with further improvements in CCTA technology in the detection of spotty calcification, more studies are needed to confirm its clinical application as a reliable feature for predicting vulnerable plaques.

4.4 Limitations and Future Directions

The above-mentioned four plaque features have been discussed with regard to their clinical applications associated with ACS and development of major adverse cardiac events. There is a growing body of evidence in the literature to show the predictive value of CCTA-derived quantitative assessment of plaque morphological features for the prediction of cardiac events.[112–116] Tesche and colleagues in their recent studies performed quantitative analysis of coronary plaque features based on CCTA in patients presented with ACS with the control group consisting of same number but stable CAD patients. A combination of Framingham risk score (area under the ROC curve-AUC = 0.54) with plaque features such as napkin-ring sign (AUC = 0.71) or remodeling index or lesion length (AUC = 0.82) significantly improved the predictive value of ACS by CCTA, with the highest predictive value achieved when the Framingham risk was combined with all of these features (AUC = 0.92) ($p < 0.05$). On a per-lesion and per-patient level assessment, these plaque markers as quantitatively assessed by CCTA were found to be significantly differently in patients with ACS when compared with the control group ($p < 0.05$).[115,116]

A multicenter study from the ROMICAT-II trial has also demonstrated the predictive value of plaque features for the prediction of major cardiac events.[117] A total of 472 patients from 9 hospitals with chest pain presenting to the emergency department were enrolled in this study. All of these four plaque features were analyzed by CCTA and compared between patients with ACS and without ACS (Fig. 4.4). All high-risk plaque features were often seen in patients with ACS compared with those without ACS ($p < 0.001$). Results showed that CCTA-derived high-risk plaque features had a direct association with ACS, but independent of significant CAD and conventional clinical risk assessment.[117]

Some of the limitations in the current studies need to be addressed by further research. One of the limitations is due to retrospective nature in most of the studies, therefore, prospectively designed cohort studies are strongly encouraged. Another limitation is the low number of ACS or cardiac events as highlighted by Puchner et al.[117] Less than 10% of the cases ($n = 37$) developed ACS when compared to those without ACS ($n = 435$). Not all of the ruptured plaques result in ACS as some of them are clinically silent. This suggests that multiple factors are involved in the development of ACS from a ruptured plaque rather than the CT assessment of morphological features of vulnerable plaque.[118] Further studies based on a large number of patients, with longer follow-up are required to determine incremental value of high-risk plaques for the prediction of ACS.

4.5 Summary and Conclusion

With rapid developments in CT image techniques, CCTA has the ability to not only reliably diagnose coronary stenosis, but also to quantitatively assess plaque morphological features with clinical evidence showing strong association with the development of major cardiac events. CCTA allows evaluation of high-risk plaque features including low-attenuation plaque, positive remodeling index, napkin-ring sign and spotty calcification. This enables assessment of individual plaques by CCTA to identify patients at potential risk of developing an ACS or major cardiac events.

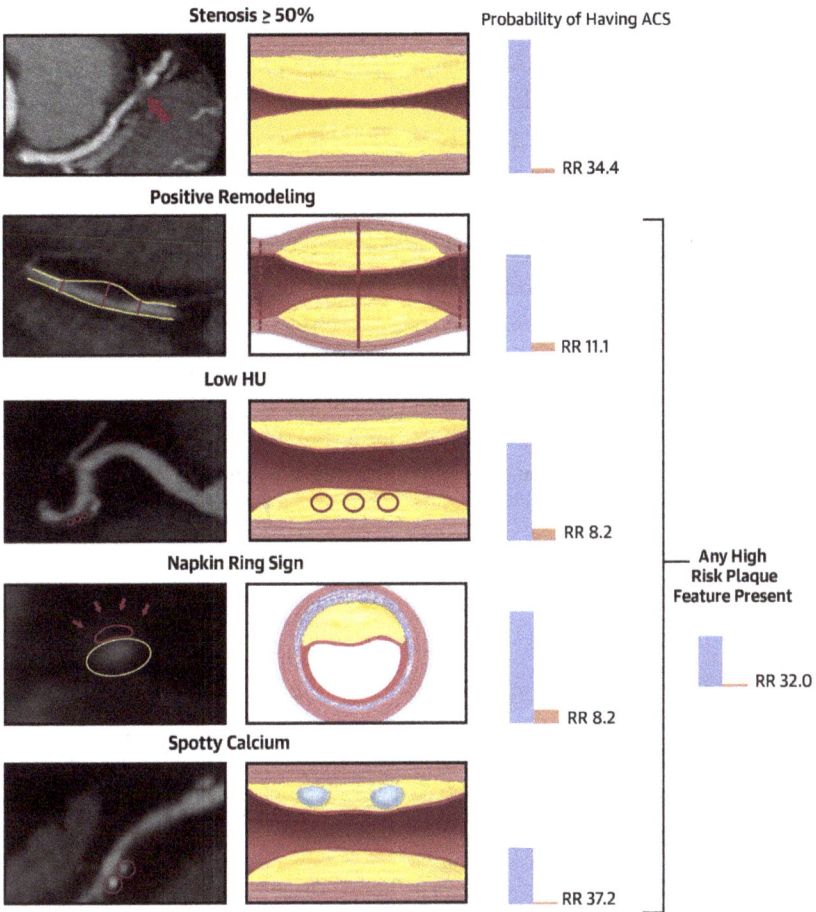

Figure 4.4. Significant stenosis and high-risk coronary plaque features and their association with the probability of ACS during index hospitalization. The two dotted red lines+ demonstrate the vessel diameters at the proximal and distal references (both 1.8 mm), and the solid red line demonstrates the maximal vessel diameter in the mid portion of the plaque (2.7 mm). The remodeling index is 1.5. Low-attenuation plaque with low HU: partially calcified plaque in the mid RCA with low <30 HU plaque. The red circles refer to the three regions of interest, with mean CT numbers of 22 HU, 19 HU, and 20 HU. Napkin-ring sign: plaque with napkin-ring sign in the mid left anterior descending coronary artery. Schematic cross-sectional view of the napkin-ring sign. The red line demonstrates the central low HU area of the plaque adjacent to the lumen (yellow ellipse) surrounded by a peripheral rim of the higher CT attenuation (red arrows). Spotty calcium: partially calcified plaque in the mid RCA with spotty calcification (diameter <3 mm in all directions; red circles). RR-relative risk. Reprinted with permission from Puchner et al.[117]

Despite significant improvements in spatial resolution, CCTA is still limited in differentiation of some plaque features, in particular, visualization of fibrous components or detection of thin-cap fibroatheroma as compared to IVUS or OCT. Another rapidly developed area of CCTA is the ability of providing functional/or physiological analysis of plaque characteristics because not all of the ACS is due to significant coronary stenosis or plaque rupture.[119] The visual assessment of lumen stenosis has been reported to correlate poorly with hemodynamic significance, particularly for intermediate stenosis between 30% and 70%.[110] The current imaging paradigm for CCTA diagnosis of CAD is based on the detailed analysis of plaque characteristics and myocardial ischemia, in addition to the lumen stenosis.[115] Therefore, investigation of hemodynamic effects of coronary plaques by CCTA represents the current research focus to identify patient-specific ischemic lesions.[120–125] CCTA-derived flow dynamics and fractional flow reserve will be discussed in Chapters 5 and 6.

References

1. Budoff MJ, Dowe D, Jollis JG et al. (2008) Diagnostic performance of 64-multidetector row coronary computed tomographic angiography for evaluation of coronary artery stenosis in individuals without known coronary artery disease: results from the prospective multicenter ACCURACY (Assessment by Coronary Computed Tomographic Angiography of Individuals Undergoing Invasive Coronary Angiography) trial. *J Am Coll Cardiol* **52**: 1724–1732.
2. Miller JM, Rochitte CE, Dewey M et al. (2008) Diagnostic performance of coronary angiography by 64-row CT. *N Engl J Med* **359**: 2324–2336.
3. Meijboom WB, Meijs MF, Schuijf JD et al. (2008) Diagnostic accuracy of 64-slice computed tomography coronary angiography: a prospective, multicenter, multivendor study. *J Am Coll Cardiol* **52**: 2135–2144.
4. Sun Z, Choo GH, Ng KH. (2012) Coronary CT angiography: current status and continuing challenges. *Br J Radiol* **85**: 495–510.
5. Xu L, Yang L, Fan Z et al. (2011) Diagnostic performance of 320-detector CT coronary angiography in patients atrial fibrillation. *Eur Radiol* **21**: 936–943.
6. Flohr TG, De Cecco CN, Schmidt B et al. (2015) Computed tomographic assessment of coronary artery disease: state-of-the-art imaging techniques. *Radiol Clin N Am* **53**: 271–285.
7. Saremi F, Achenbach S. (2015) Coronary plaque characterization using CT. *AJR Am J Roentegenol* **204**: W249–W260.

8. Henzler T, Porubsky S, Kayed H *et al.* (2011) Attenuation-based characterization of coronary atherosclerotic plaque: comparison of dual source and dual energy CT with single-source CT and histopathology. *Eur J Radiol* **80**: 54–59.
9. Marwan M, Taher MA, El Meniawy K *et al.* (2011) In vivo CT detection of lipid-rich coronary artery atherosclerotic plaques using quantitative histogram analysis: a head to head comparison with IVUS. *Atherosclerosis* **215**: 110–115.
10. Pundziute G, Schuijf JD, Jukema JW *et al.* (2008) Head-to-head comparison of coronary plaque evaluation between multislice computed tomography and intravascular ultrasound radiofrequency data analysis. *JACC Cardiovasc Interv* **1**: 176–182.
11. Lin F, Shaw LJ, Berman DS *et al.* (2008) Multidetector computed tomography coronary artery plaque predictors of stress-induced myocardial ischemia by SPECT. *Atherosclerosis* **197**: 700–709.
12. Pundziute G, Schuijf JD, Jukema JW *et al.* (2007) Prognostic value of multislice computed tomography coronary angiography in patients with known or suspected coronary artery disease. *J Am Coll Cardiol* **49**: 62–70.
13. van Werkhoven JM, Schuijf JD, Gaemperli O *et al.* (2009) Prognostic value of multislice computed tomography and gated single-photon emission computed tomography in patients with suspected coronary artery disease. *J Am Coll Cardiol* **53**: 623–632.
14. Sun Z, Al Moudi M, Cao Y. (2014) CT angiography in the diagnosis of cardiovascular disease: a transformation in cardiovascular CT practice. *Quant Imaging Med Surg* **4**: 376–396.
15. Sun Z, Lin CH, Davidson R, Dong C, Liao Y. (2008) Diagnostic value of 64-slice CT angiography in coronary artery disease: a systematic review. *Eur J Radiol* **67**: 78–84.
16. Abdulla J, Abildstrom Z, Gotzsche O *et al.* (2007) 64-multislice detector computed tomography coronary angiography as potential alternative to conventional coronary angiography: a systematic review and meta-analysis. *Eur Heart J* **28**: 3042–3050.
17. Stein PD, Yaekoub AY, Matta F, Sostman HD. (2008) 64-slice CT for diagnosis of coronary artery disease: a systematic review. *Am J Med* **121**: 715–725.
18. Mowatt G, Cook JA, Hillis GS *et al.* (2008) 64-slice computed tomography angiography in the diagnosis and assessment of coronary artery disease: systematic review and meta-analysis. *Heart* **94**: 1386–1393.
19. Guo SL, Guo YM, Zhai YN *et al.* (2011) Diagnostic accuracy of first generation dual-source computed tomography in the assessment of coronary artery disease: a meta-analysis from 24 studies. *Int J Cardiovasc Imaging* **27**: 755–771.
20. Salavati A, Radmanesh F, Heidari K *et al.* (2012) Dual-source computed tomography angiography for diagnosis and assessment of coronary artery disease: systematic review and meta-analysis. *J Cardiovasc Comput Tomogr* **6**: 78–90.
21. Gaudio C, Pellicia F, Evangelista A *et al.* (2013) 320-row computed tomography angiography vs conventional coronary angiography in patients with suspected coronary artery disease: a systematic review and meta-analysis. *Int J Cardiol* **168**: 1562–1564.

22. Li S, Ni Q, Wu H *et al.* (2013) Diagnostic accuracy of 320-slice computed tomography angiography for detection of coronary artery stenosis: Meta-analysis. *Int J Cardiol* **168**: 2699–2705.

23. Sun Z, Lin C. (2014) Diagnostic value of 320-slice coronary CT angiography in coronary artery disease: a systematic review and meta-analysis. *Curr Med Imaging Rev* **10**: 272–280.

24. Sun Z. (2013) Comment on: Diagnostic accuracy of 320-slice computed tomography angiography for detection of coronary artery stenosis: meta-analysis. *Int J Cardiol* **168**: 4895–4896.

25. Funabashi N, Namihira Y, Irie R *et al.* (2016) Recommended acquisition parameters in achieving successful evaluation of coronary lumen patency surrounded by XIENCE of diameter <3.0 mm in 2nd-generation 320-slice CT. XIENCE phantom study part 2. *Int J Cardiol* **202**: 541–545.

26. Chen MY, Shanbhag SM, Arai AE. (2013) Submillisievert median radiation dose for coronary angiography with a second-generation 320-detector row CT scanner in 107 consecutive patients. *Radiology* **267**: 76–85.

27. Ghekiere O, Nchimi A, Djekic J *et al.* (2016) Coronary computed tomography angiography: patient-related factors determining image quality using a second-generation 320-slice CT scanner. *Int J Cardiol* **221**: 970–976.

28. Bamberg F, Abbara S, Schlett CL *et al.* (2010) Predictors of image quality of coronary computed tomography in the acute care setting of patients with chest pain. *Eur J Radiol* **74**: 182–188.

29. Muenzel D, Noel PB, Dorn F, Dobritz M, Rummeny EJ, Huber A. (2011) Step and shoot coronary CT angiography using 256-slice CT: effect of heart rate and heart rate variability on image quality. *Eur Radiol* **21**: 2277–2284.

30. Stolzmann P, Goetti RP, Maurovich-Horvat P *et al.* (2011) Predictors of image quality in high-pitch coronary CT angiography. *AJR Am J Roentgenol* **197**: 851–858.

31. Meinel FG, Canstein C, Schoepf UJ *et al.* (2014) Image quality and radiation dose of low tube voltage 3rd generation dual-source coronary CT angiography in obese patients: a phantom study. *Eur Radiol* **24**: 1643–1650.

32. Gordic S, Husarik D, Desbiolles L *et al.* (2014) High-pitch coronary CT angiography with third generation dual-source CT: limits of heart rate. *Int J Cardiovasc Imaging* **30**: 1173–1179.

33. Gordic S, Desbiolles L, Sedimair M *et al.* (2016) Optimizing radiation dose by using advanced modelled iterative reconstruction in high-pitch coronary CT angiography. *Eur Radiol* **26**: 459–468.

34. Mangold S, Wichmann JL, Schoepf UJ *et al.* (2017) Diagnostic accuracy of coronary CT angiography using 3rd-generation dual-source CT and automated tube voltage selection: clinical application in a non-obese and obese patient population. *Eur Radiol* **27**: 2298–2308.

35. Koplay M, Erdogan H, Avci A *et al.* (2016) Radiation dose and diagnostic accuracy of high-pitch dual-source coronary angiography in the evaluation of coronary artery stenosis. *Diagn Interv Imaging* **97**: 461–469.

36. Achenbach S, Marwan M, Ropers D *et al.* (2010) Coronary computed tomography angiography with a consistent dose below 1 mSv using prospectively electrocardiogram-triggered high-pitch spiral acquisition. *Eur Heart J* **31**: 340–346.

37. Layritz C, Schmid J, Achenbach S *et al.* (2014) Accuracy of prospectively ECG-triggered very low-dose coronary dual-source CT angiography using iterative reconstruction for the detection of coronary artery disease: comparison with invasive catheterization. *Eur Heart J Cardiovasc Imaging* **15**: 1238–1245.

38. Eisentopf J, Achenbach S, Ulzheimer S *et al.* (2013) Low-dose dual-source CT angiography wit iterative reconstruction for coronary artery stent evaluation. *JACC Cardiovasc Imaging* **6**: 458–465.

39. Schuhbaeck A, Achenbach S, Layritz C *et al.* (2013) Image quality of ultra-low radiation exposure coronary CT angiography with an effective dose <0.1 mSv using high-pitch spiral acquisition and raw data-based iterative reconstruction. *Eur Radiol* **23**: 597–606.

40. Stehli J, Fuchs TA, Bull S *et al.* (2014) Accuracy of coronary CT angiography using a submillisievert fraction of radiation exposure: comparison with invasive coronary angiography. *J Am Coll Cardiol* **64**: 772–780.

41. Ellis S, Alderman E, Cain K, Fisher L, Sanders W, Bourassa M. (1998) Prediction of risk of anterior myocardial infarction by lesion severity and measurement method of stenoses in the left anterior descending coronary distribution: a CASS Registry Study. *J Am Coll Cardiol* **11**: 908–916.

42. Stone GW, Maehara A, Lansky AJ *et al.* (2011) A prospective natural history study of coronary atherosclerosis. *N Engl J Med* **364**: 226–235.

43. Virmani R, Kolodgie FD, Burke AP, Farb A, Schwartz SM. (2000) Lessons from sudden coronary death: a comprehensive morphological classification scheme for atherosclerotic lesions. *Arterioscler Thromb Vasc Biol* **20**: 1262–1275.

44. Virmani R, Burke AP, Farb A, Kolodgie FD. (2006) Pathology of the vulnerable plaque. *J Am Coll Cardiol* **47**: C13–C18.

45. Jia H, Abtahian F, Aguirre AD *et al.* (2013) In vivo diagnosis of plaque erosion and calcified nodule in patients with acute coronary syndrome by intravascular optical coherence tomography. *J Am Coll Cardiol* **62**: 1748–1758.

46. Maurovich-Horvat P, Ferencik M, Voros S, Merkely B, Hoffmann U. (2014) Comprehensive plaque assessment by coronary CT angiography. *Nat Rev Cardiol* **11**: 390–402.

47. Nadjiri J, Hausleiter J, Jahnichen C *et al.* (2016) Incremental prognostic value of quantitative plaque assessment in coronary CT angiography during 5 years of follow-up. *J Cardiovasc Comput Tomogr* **10**: 97–104.

48. Psaltis PJ, Nicholls SJ. (2016) Focusing light on the vulnerable plaque. *Nat Rev Cardiol* **13**: 253–255.

49. Hecht HS, Achenbach S, Kondo T, Narula J. (2015) High risk plaque features on coronary CT angiography. *JACC Cardiovasc Imaging* **8**: 1336–1339.

50. Kopp AF, Schroeder S, Baumbach A *et al.* (2011) Non-invasive characterisation of coronary lesion morphology and composition by multislice CT: first results in comparison with intracoronary ultrasound. *Eur Radiol* **11**: 1607–1611.

51. Schroeder S, Kopp Ap, Baumbach A *et al.* (2001) Noninvasive detection and evaluation of atherosclerotic coronary plaques with multislice computed tomography. *J Am Coll Cardiol* **37**: 1430–1435.

52. Leber AW, Knez A, Becker A *et al.* (2004) Accuracy of multidetector spiral computed tomography in identifying and differentiating the composition of coronary atherosclerotic plaques: a comparative study with intracoronary ultrasound. *J Am Coll Cardiol* **43**: 1241–1247.

53. Pohle K, Achenbach S, Macneill B *et al.* (2007) Characterization of non-calcified coronary atherosclerotic plaque by multi-detector row CT: comparison to IVUS. *Atherosclerosis* **190**: 174–180.

54. Becker CR, Nikolaou K, Muders M *et al.* (2003) *Ex vivo* coronary atherosclerotic plaque characterization with multi-detector-row CT. *Eur Radiol* **13**: 2094–2098.

55. Gauss S, Achenbach S, Pflederer T, Schuhback A, Daniel WG, Marwan M. (2011) Assessment of coronary artery remodelling by dual-source CT: a head-to-head comparison with intravascular ultrasound. *Heart* **97**: 991–997.

56. Takaoka H, Ishibashi I, Uehara M, Rubin GD, Komuro I, Funabashi N. (2012) Comparison of image characteristics of plaques in culprit coronary arteries by 64 slice CT and intravascular ultrasound in acute coronary syndromes. *Int J Cardiol* **160**: 119–126.

57. Motoyama S, Kondo T, Sarai M *et al.* (2007) Multislice computed tomographic characteristics of coronary lesions in acute coronary syndromes. *J Am Coll Cardiol* **50**: 319–326.

58. Motoyama S, Sarai M, Harigaya H *et al.* (2009) Computed tomographic angiography characteristics of atherosclerotic plaques subsequently resulting in acute coronary syndrome. *J Am Coll Cardiol* 54: 49–57.

59. Vazquez-Figueroa JG, Rinehart S, Qian Z *et al.* (2013) Prospective validation that vulnerable plaque associated with major adverse outcomes have large plaque volume, less dense calcium, and more non-calcified plaque by quantitative, three-dimensional measurements using intravascular ultrasound with radiofrequency backscatter analysis. Results from the ATLANTA I Study. *J Cardiovasc Trans Res* **6**: 762–771.

60. Achenbach S, Friedrich MG, Nagel E *et al.* (2013) CV Imaging: What was new in 2012? *JACC Cardiovasc. Imaging* **6**: 714–734.

61. Nishio M, Ueda Y, Matsuo K *et al.* (2011) Detection of disrupted plaques by coronary CT: comparison with angioscopy. *Heart* **97**: 1397–1402.

62. Cademartiri E, Mollet NR, Runza G *et al.* (2005) Influence of intracoronary attenuation on coronary plaque measurements using multislice computed tomography: observation in an ex vivo model of coronary computed tomography angiography. *Eur Radiol* **15**: 1426–1431.

63. Shmilovich H, Cheng VY, Tamarappoo BK *et al.* (2011) Vulnerable plaque features on coronary CT angiography as markers of inducible regional myocardial hypoperfusion from severe coronary artery stenosis. *Atherosclerosis* **219**: 588–595.

64. Kristando W, van Ooijen PM, Jansen-van der Weide MC, Vliegenhart R, Oudkerk M. (2013) A meta-analysis and hierarchical classification of HU-based atherosclerotic plaque characterization criteria. *PLOS One* **8**: e73460.

65. Kubo T, Maehara A, Mintz GS *et al.* (2010) The dynamic nature of coronary artery lesion morphology assessed by serial virtual histology intravascular ultrasound tissue characterization. *J Am Coll Cardiol* **55**: 1590–1597.

66. Pflederer T, Marwan M, Schepis T *et al.* (2010) Characterization of culprit lesions in acute coronary syndrome using coronary dual-source CT angiography. *Atherosclerosis* **211**: 437–444.

67. Narula J, Strauss HW. (2007) The popcorn plaques. *Nat Med* **13**: 532–534.

68. Glagov S, Weisenberg E, Zarins CK, Stankunavicius R, Kolettis GJ. (1987) Compensatory enlargement of human atherosclerotic coronary arteries. *N Engl J Med* **316**: 1371–1375.

69. Nishioka T, Luo H, Eigler NL, Berglund H, Kim C, Siegel RJ. (1996) Contribution of inadequate compensatory enlargement to development of human coronary artery stenosis: an in vitro intravascular ultrasound study. *J Am Coll Cardiol* **27**: 1571–1576.

70. Sun Z, Lei Xu. (2014) Coronary CT angiography in the quantitative assessment of coronary plaques. *Biomed Res Int* **2014**: 346380.

71. Varnava AM, Mills PG, Davies MJ. (2002) Relationship between coronary artery remodeling and plaque vulnerability. *Circulation* **105**: 939–943.

72. Schmid M, Pflederer T, Jang JK *et al.* (2008) Relationship between degree of remodelling and CT attenuation of plaque in coronary atherosclerotic lesions: an in vivo analysis by multi-detector computed tomography. *Atherosclerosis* **197**: 457–464.

73. Kroner ESJ, van Velzen JE, Boogers MJ *et al.* (2011) Positive remodelling on coronary computed tomography as a marker for plaque vulnerability on virtual histology intravascular ultrasound. *Am J Cardiol* **107**: 1725–1729.

74. Obaid DR, Calvert PA, Brown A *et al.* (2017) Coronary CT angiography features of ruptured and high-risk atherosclerotic plaques: Correlation with intra-vascular ultrasound. *J Cardiovasc Comput Tomogr* **11**(6): 455–461.

75. Mintz G S, Nissen SE, Anderson WD *et al.* (2001) American College of Cardiology clinical expert consensus document on standards for acquisition, measurement and reporting of intravascular ultrasound studies (IVUS). A report of the American College of Cardiology Task Force on clinical expert consensus documents. *J Am Coll Cardiol* **37**: 1478–1492.

76. Kashiwagi M, Tanaka A, Kitabata H *et al.* (2009) Feasibility of noninvasive assessment of thin-cap fibroatheroma by multidetector computed tomography. *JACC Cardiovasc Imaging* **2**: 1412–1419.

77. Ito T, Terashima M, Kaneda H *et al.* (2011) Comparison of in vivo assessment of vulnerable plaque by 64-slice multislice computed tomography versus optical coherence tomography. *Am J Cardiol* **107**: 1270–1277.

78. Kim SY, Kim KS, Seung MJ *et al.* (2010) The culprit lesion score on multi-detector computed tomography can detect vulnerable coronary artery plaque. *Int J Cardiovasc Imaging* **26** (Suppl. 2): 245–252.

79. Kitagawa T, Yamamoto H, Horiguchi J *et al.* (2009) Characterization of noncalcified coronary plaques and identification of culprit lesions in patients with acute coronary syndrome by 64-slice computed tomography. *JACC Cardiovasc Imaging* **2**: 153–160.

80. Conte E, Annoni A, Pontone G *et al.* (2017) Evaluation of coronary plaque characteristics with coronary computed tomography angiography in patients with non-obstructive coronary artery disease: a long-term follow-up study. *Eur Heart J Cardiovasc Imaging* **18**: 1170–1178.

81. Achenbach S, Ropers D, Hoffmann U *et al.* (2004) Assessment of coronary remodeling in stenotic and nonstenotic coronary atherosclerotic lesions by multidetector spiral computed tomography. *J Am Coll Cardiol* **43**: 842–847.

82. Hoffmann U, Moselewski F, Nieman K *et al.* (2006) Noninvasive assessment of plaque morphology and composition in culprit and stable lesions in acute coronary syndrome and stable lesions in stable angina by multidetector computed tomography. *J Am Coll Cardiol* **47**: 1655–1662.

83. Narula J, Achenbach S. (2009) Napkin-ring necrotic cores: defining circumferential extent of necrotic cores in unstable plaques. *JACC Cardiovasc Imaging* **2**: 1436–1438.

84. Maurovich-Horvat P, Schlett CL, Alkadhi H *et al.* (2012) The napkin-ring sign indicates advanced atherosclerotic lesions in coronary CT angiography. *JACC Cardiovasc Imaging* **5**: 1243–1252.

85. Kodama T, Kondo T, Oida A, Fujimoto S, Narula J. (2012) Computed tomographic angiography-verified plaque characteristics and slow-flow phenomenon during percutaneous coronary intervention. *JACC Cardiovasc Interv* **5**: 636–643.

86. Maurovich-Horvat P, Hoffmann U, Vorpahl M, Nakano M, Virmani R, Alkadhi H. (2010) The napkin-ring sign: CT signature of high-risk coronary plaques? *JACC Cardiovasc Imaging* **3**: 440–444.

87. Seifarth H, Schlett CL, Nakano M *et al.* (2012) Histopathological correlates of the napkin-ring sign plaque in coronary CT angiography. *Atherosclerosis* **224**: 90–96.

88. Otsuka K, Fukuda S, Tanaka A *et al.* (2013) Napkin-ring sign on coronary CT angiography for the prediction of acute coronary syndrome. *JACC Cardiovasc Imaging* **6**: 448–457.

89. Yamamoto H, Kitagawa T, Kihara Y. (2013) Dose napkin-ring sign suggest possibility to identify rupture-prone plaque in coronary computed tomography angiography? *J Cardiol* **62**: 328–329.

90. Yang DH, Kang SJ, Koo HJ *et al.* (2017) Coronary CT angiography characteristics of OCT-defined thin-cap fibroatheroma: a section-to-section comparison study. *Eur Radiol.* doi: 10.1007/s00330-017-4992-8.

91. Liu T, Maurovich-Horvat P, Mayrhofer T *et al.* (2017) Quantitative coronary plaque analysis predicts high-risk plaque morphology on coronary computed tomography

angiography: results from the ROMICAT II trial. *Int J Cardiovasc Imaging*. doi: 10.1007/s10554-017-1228-6.

92. Rumberger JA, Simons DB, Fitzpatrick LA *et al.* (1995) Coronary artery calcium area by electron-beam computed tomography and coronary atherosclerotic plaque area. A histopathologic correlative study. *Circulation* **92**: 2157–2162.

93. Baumgart D, Schmermund A, Goerge G *et al.* (1997) Comparison of electron beam computed tomography with intracoronary ultrasound and coronary angiography for detection of coronary atherosclerosis. *J Am Coll Cardiol* **30**: 57–64.

94. Kajinami K, Seki H, Takekoshi N, Mabuchi H. (1997) Coronary calcification and coronary atherosclerosis: site by site comparative morphologic study of electron beam computed tomography and coronary angiography. *J Am Coll Cardiol* **29**: 1549–1556.

95. Alluri K, Joshi PH, Henry TS, Blumenthal RS, Nasir K, Blaha MJ. (2015) Scoring of coronary artery calcium scans: history, assumptions, current limitations, and future directions. *Atherosclerosis* **239**: 109–117.

96. Rana JS, Gransar H, Wong ND *et al.* (2012) Comparative value of coronary artery calcium and multiple blood biomarkers for prognostication of cardiovascular events. *Am J Cardiol* **109**: 1449–1453.

97. Gottlieb I, Miller JM, Arbab-Zadeh A *et al.* (2010) The absence of coronary calcification does not exclude obstructive coronary artery disease or the need for revascularization in patients referred for conventional coronary angiography. *J Am Coll Cardiol* **55**: 627–634.

98. Budoff MJ, Nasir K, McClelland RL *et al.* (2009) Coronary calcium predicts events better with absolute calcium scores than age-sex-race/ethnicity percentiles: MESA (Multi-Ethnic Study of Atherosclerosis). *J Am Coll Cardiol* **53**: 345–352.

99. Taylor AJ, Bindeman J, Feuerstein I *et al.* (2005) Coronary calcium independently predicts incident premature coronary heart disease over measured cardiovascular risk factors: mean three-year outcomes in the Prospective Army Coronary Calcium (PACC) project. *J Am Coll Cardiol* **46**: 807–814.

100. LaMonte MJ, FitzGerald SJ, Church TS *et al.* (2005) Coronary artery calcium score and coronary heart disease events in a large cohort of asymptomatic men and women. *Am J Epidemiol* **162**: 421–429.

101. Goldstein JA, Chinnaiyan KM, Abidov A *et al.* (2011) The CT-STAT (Coronary computed tomographic angiography for systematic triage of acute chest pain patients to treatment) trial. *J Am Coll Cardiol* **58**: 1414–1422.

102. Alexanderson E, Canseco-Leon N, Inarra F, Meave A, Dey D. (2012) Prognostic value of cardiovascular CT: is coronary artery calcium screening enough? The added value of CCTA. *J Nucl Cardiol* **19**: 601–608.

103. Hartaigh BO, Valenti V, Cho I *et al.* (2016) 15-year prognostic utility of coronary artery calcium scoring for all-cause mortality in the elderly. *Atherosclerosis* **246**: 361–366.

104. Johnson KM, Dowe DA, Brink JA. (2009) Traditional clinical risk assessment tools do not accurately predict coronary atherosclerotic plaque burden: a CT angiography study. *AJR Am J Roentgenol* **192**: 235–243.

105. Nicoll R, Wiklund U, Zhao Y *et al.* (2016) The coronary calcium score is a more accurate predictor of significant coronary stenosis than conventional risk factors in symptomatic patients: Euro-CCAD study. *Int J Cardiol* **207**: 13–19.

106. Huang H, Virmani R, Younis H, Burke AP, Kamm RD, Lee RT. (2001) The impact of calcification on the biomechanical stability of atherosclerotic plaques. *Circulation* **103**: 1051–1056.

107. Maldonado N, Kelly-Arnold A, Vengrenyuk Y *et al.* (2012) A mechanistic analysis of the role of microcalcifications in atherosclerotic plaque stability: potential implications for plaque rupture. *Am J Physiol Heart Circ Physiol* **303**: H619–H628.

108. Mauriello A, Servadei F, Zoccai GB *et al.* (2013) Coronary calcification identifies the vulnerable patient rather than the vulnerable plaque. *Atherosclerosis* **229**: 124–129.

109. Kataoka Y, Wolski K, Uno K *et al.* (2012) Spotty calcification as a marker of accelerated progression of coronary atherosclerosis: insights from serial intravascular ultrasound. *J Am Coll Cardiol* **59**: 1592–1597.

110. Ehara S, Kobayashi Y, Yoshiyama M *et al.* (2004) Spotty calcification typifies the culprit plaque in patients with acute myocardial infarction: an intravascular ultrasound study. *Circulation* **110**: 3424–3429.

111. Otsuka F, Finn AV, Virmani R. (2013) Do vulnerable and ruptured plaques hide in heavily calcified arteries? *Atherosclerosis* **229**: 34–37.

112. Min JK, Feignoux J, Treutenaere J, Laperche T, Sablayrolles J. (2010) The prognostic value of multidetector coronary CT angiography for the prediction of major adverse cardiovascular events: a multicenter observational cohort study. *Int J Cardiovasc Imaging* **26**: 721–728.

113. Cheruvu C, Precious B, Naoum C *et al.* (2016) Long term prognostic utility of coronary CT angiography in patients with no modifiable coronary artery disease risk factors: results from the 5 year follow-up of the CONFIRM International Multicenter Registry. *J Cardiovasc Comput Tomogr* **10**: 22–27.

114. Szilveszter B, Celeng C, Maurovich-Horvat P (2016) Plaque assessment by coronary CT. *Int J Cardiovasc Imaging* **32**(1): 161–72.

115. Tesche C, Plank F, De Cecco CN *et al.* (2016) Prognostic implications of coronary CT angiography-derived quantitative markers for the prediction of major adverse cardiac events. *J Cardiovasc Comput Tomogr* **10**: 458–465.

116. Tesche C, Caruso D, De Cecco CN *et al.* (2017) Coronary computed tomography angiography-derived plaque quantification in patients with acute coronary syndrome. *Am J Cardiol* **119**: 712–718.

117. Puchner SB, Liu T, Mayrhofer T *et al.* (2014) High-risk plaque detected on coronary CT angiography predicts acute coronary syndromes independent of significant stenosis in acute chest pain: results from the ROMICAT-II trial. *J Am Coll Cardiol* **64**: 684–692.

118. Yoo SM, Lee HY, Jin KN *et al.* (2017) Current concepts of vulnerable plaque on coronary CT angiography. *Cardiovasc Imaging Asia* **1**: 4–12.

119. Kanwar S, Stone GW, Singh M *et al.* (2016) Acute coronary syndromes without coronary plaque rupture. *Nat Rev Cardiol* **13**: 257–265.

120. Tonino PA, De Bryune B, Pijls NH *et al.* (2009) Fractional flow reserve versus angiography for guiding percutaneous coronary intervention. *N Engl J Med* **360**: 213–224.

121. Dweck MR, Doris MK, Motwani M *et al.* (2016) Imaging of coronary atherosclerosis-evolution towards new treatment strategies. *Nat Rev Cardiol* **13**: 533–548.

122. Kim HJ, Vignon-Clementel IE, Coogan JS, Figueroa CA, Jansen KE, Taylor CA. (2010) Patient-specific modeling of blood flow and pressure in human coronary arteries. *Ann Biomed Eng* **38**: 3195–3209.

123. Taylor CA, Fonte TA, Min JK. (2013) Computational fluid dynamics applied to cardiac computed tomography for noninvasive quantification of fractional flow reserve: scientific basis. *J Am Coll Cardiol* **61**: 2233–2241.

124. Nieman K, de Feijter PJ. (2013) Aerodynamics in cardiac CT. *Circ. Cardiovasc Imaging* **6**: 853–854.

125. Ramkumar PG, Mitsouras D, Feldman CL, Stone PH, Rybicki FJ. (2009) New advances in cardiac computed tomography. *Curr Opin Cardiol* **24**: 596–603.

5 Coronary CT Angiography-Derived Computational Fluid Dynamics

Abstract

Computational fluid dynamics (CFD) is a numerical method that is widely used in mechanical engineering. In recent years, there has been a growing interest in the investigation of cardiovascular disease with use of CFD simulations. Coronary computed tomography angiography (CCTA)-derived CFD simulations are increasingly used to study the local flow fields and hemodynamic changes in relation to the development of atherosclerosis and plaque progression to rupture-prone plaques. Of these applications, the use of CFD to identify risk factors for plaque formation, in particular, to detect vulnerable or high-risk plaques represents an important clinical application. This chapter provides an overview of the CFD applications in coronary artery disease (CAD), with a focus on CCTA-derived CFD applications in CAD in terms of wall shear stress and vulnerable plaque analysis.

Keywords: coronary artery disease, computational fluid dynamics, coronary computed tomography angiography, hemodynamics, plaque.

5.1 Introduction

In recent years, investigation of hemodynamic changes in the coronary artery system has gained a lot of interest for studying atherosclerosis and plaque formation.[1,2] The role of blood flow in atherosclerosis is due to the fact that inflammatory change and plaque formation are usually noticed near side branches or the bifurcation area, where blood flow is non-uniform and disturbed, thus influencing the behavior of endothelial cells (ECs).[3,4] Of various hemodynamic parameters, wall shear stress (WSS) is the most important parameter which has significant impact on both morphological alterations and physiological changes of ECs.

WSS is determined by blood flow and is defined as the frictional force exerted by blood flow on the endothelial surface of the arterial wall. WSS changes with the geometric environment of an anatomical location, with high WSS observed at the outer curvature and low WSS at the inner curvature of the arterial wall.[5,6] The magnitude of WSS (expressed as Pascal — Pa: $1 \text{ Pa} = 1 \text{ N/m}^2 = 10 \text{ dynes/cm}^2$) is also determined by the blood flow velocity. WSS is significantly increased at the region of significant coronary stenosis caused by atherosclerotic plaque due to acceleration of blood flow through narrowed cross-sectional area (Fig. 5.1).[7]

In vivo estimation of WSS can be performed through computational fluid dynamics (CFD) simulations. CFD is a numerical method that calculates flow fields of liquids within a structure or the reconstructed arterial volume for solving fluid dynamics.[8] To perform CFD simulations, several factors need to be defined, including generation of an accurate 3D geometry of the coronary artery tree using imaging data, mainly from coronary computed tomography angiographic (CCTA) images; physiological parameters to simulate blood flow in terms of flow velocity and pressure

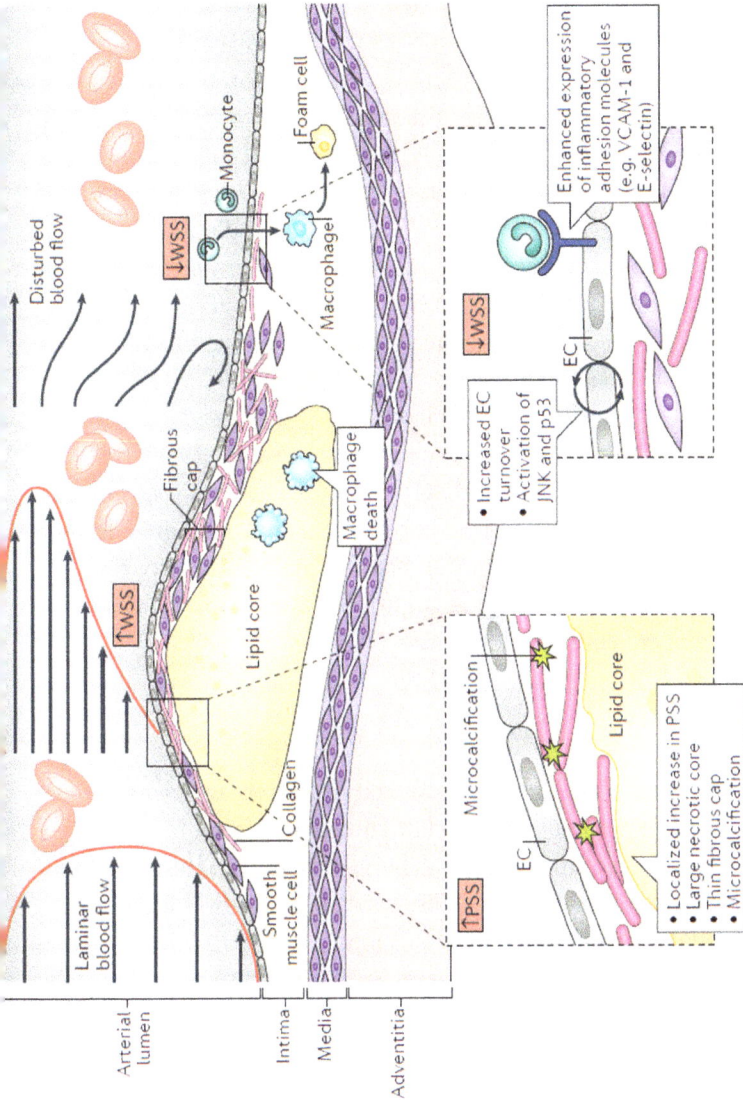

Figure 5.1. Biomechanical forces in atherosclerosis. Changes in both WSS and plaque structural stress (PSS) play important roles in coronary plaque development, progression and rupture. Geometrical changes to the arterial lumen induce alterations in blood flow that result in low WSS regions, which induce the expression of inflammatory adhesion molecules and modify EC turnover. In established atherosclerotic lesions, subtle changes in plaque composition and/or architecture increase PSS, making the plaque more vulnerable to rupture. JNK: c-Jun N-terminal kinases; p53: cellular tumor antigen p53; VCAM-1: vascular cell adhesion molecule 1. Reprinted with permission from Brown et al.[9]

through coronary arteries; and numerical solutions for calculation of motion and behavior of blood flow inside the coronary arteries.[9] These comprise the basic elements for estimating WSS and studying the hemodynamic changes in coronary artery disease (CAD).

There have been an increasing number of studies available in the literature with regard to the use of 3D reconstruction of coronary artery tree with numerical simulation using CFD techniques based on idealized or patient-specific coronary models to study hemodynamics inside the coronary arteries.[10–16] Intravascular ultrasound (IVUS) is the gold standard for quantitative assessment of plaque features, and CFD simulations based on IVUS images have been well correlated to WSS changes and atherosclerosis development, and coronary plaque progression in terms of plaque component changes.[17–23] However, due to the invasive nature of IVUS, this technique is not widely available in clinical practice. Currently, more studies are focusing on the CFD analysis of CAD based on CCTA-generated 3D reconstruction of coronary models. This chapter provides an overview of CCTA-derived CFD applications in CAD with a focus on the evidence-based review of the CFD in the biomechanics of atherosclerotic plaques and in the detection of high-risk plaques and plaque progression, thus achieving the goal of identifying high-risk patients for the development of major adverse cardiac events.

5.2 Overview of CFD

The value of CFD lies in developing new and improved devices and system designs through computational simulations resulting in enhanced efficiency and lower operating costs.[16] The governing equations of fluid dynamics can be computed to acquire coronary blood flow and pressure, which are essential for generating accurate simulation results. These equations, namely, Navier–Stokes equations, have been in use for more than 100 years. In order to perform simulation of realistic coronary blood flow, a domain of interest must be defined, and boundary conditions specified because these represent the necessary steps for CFD simulations in the coronary arteries.

For geometric reconstruction and generation of 3D coronary artery model, both fluid and structural domains of vessel surfaces are meshed with triangles comprising hexahedral cells with the aim of minimizing numerical diffusion and lowering the number of elements. Reliable hemodynamic parameters in the normal coronary arteries are required for a CFD study, and this can be obtained with imaging techniques such as Doppler ultrasound or phase-contrast magnetic resonance imaging (MRI).[24,25] Blood flow in the coronary artery is unsteady due to variation of flow associated with the cardiac cycle. Most of the studies take the approach to apply the cardiac cycle at the main aorta to provide both the inflow and outflow conditions. The inlet and outlet boundary conditions are defined based on a physiological flow rate and pressure at the aorta.[26] A pulsatile flow of the blood is simulated and imposed at the inlet of the coronary artery by assigning a flow profile equal to the peak velocity/pressure measured at each point in the cardiac cycle. A prescribed pressure of 0 mmHg is applied at the outlet of the coronary artery.[27,28] This allows observation of hemodynamic changes in the arterial system including coronary artery.[29–32]

Based on the average physiological human coronary flow data that are reported in the literature, the average blood flow into the left coronary artery is 57 mL/min, reaching a maximum value of 105 mL/min during the diastolic phases, while the mass flow rate for the right coronary artery is 112.9 mL/min.[33,34] The blood flow distribution in the left coronary artery is calculated as 71% directed through the left anterior descending (LAD) and 29% through left circumflex (LCx) arteries according to the literature.[33,35]

Since blood flow to coronary artery varies during cardiac cycles, a flow simulation is conducted over a time-span of several cardiac cycles represented by time steps. These time steps can be divided into a number of coupling iterations, with each time step converged to a residual target of less than 1×10^{-4} by approximately 100 iterations.[4,36,37]

Most of the CFD simulations are based on rigid coronary models, either realistic or patient-specific geometric coronary artery models. However, the impact of blood flow on coronary artery wall changes should be considered to ensure successful simulation of blood flow and corresponding hemodynamic behavior. The fluid–structure interaction (FSI) is an approach that can simultaneously model blood flow and arterial wall deformations, and it has attracted increasing interests in recent years.[38–41] A recent study using idealized and realistic coronary models has shown significant differences between FSI and rigid models. Results showed the apparent qualitative discrepancies in WSS distributions over the bifurcation apex and the moderate narrow lumen site downstream to the LAD, and obvious quantitative differences in WSS profiles at the bifurcation apex over the diastole phase, respectively.[35] Furthermore, some specific features related to coronary artery geometry such as tortuosity or kinking also lead to flow changes, thus generating impact on the distribution of WSS.[42–44] These findings indicate that the anatomical regions in the coronary artery are prone to develop atherosclerotic lesions, which will be discussed in detail in the following sections.

5.3 Coronary CT Angiography-derived CFD Applications

Apart from WSS, which is the key hemodynamic parameter for studying atherosclerosis and coronary plaque (Fig. 5.2), other hemodynamic parameters, such as wall pressure, flow velocity, time-averaged wall shear stress (TAWSS), oscillatory shear index (OSI), and relative residence time (RRT), also contribute to the development of atherosclerosis and identification of vulnerable plaques. These hemodynamic parameters are defined as follows:

- **WSS**: A parallel hemodynamic force residing within the endothelial surface of the arterial wall.[45] It affects EC functions and plays an important role in the generation, progression and destabilization of atherosclerotic rupture-prone plaque.
- **Wall pressure**: Defined as the driving force on coronary wall at per unit area. High pressure indicates stenotic coronary lesions, and also arterial growth with aneurysmal formation in the aorta.
- **Flow velocity or flow rate**: Flow volume passing through a given surface per unit time. High flow velocity/flow rate indicates hemodynamic disturbance, which is commonly seen in stenotic regions.
- **TAWSS**: Averages the time-varying WSS over the cardiac cycle.
- **OSI**: A metric of flow reversal. It measures WSS variation due to changes in the direction of blood flow during the pulsatile cardiac

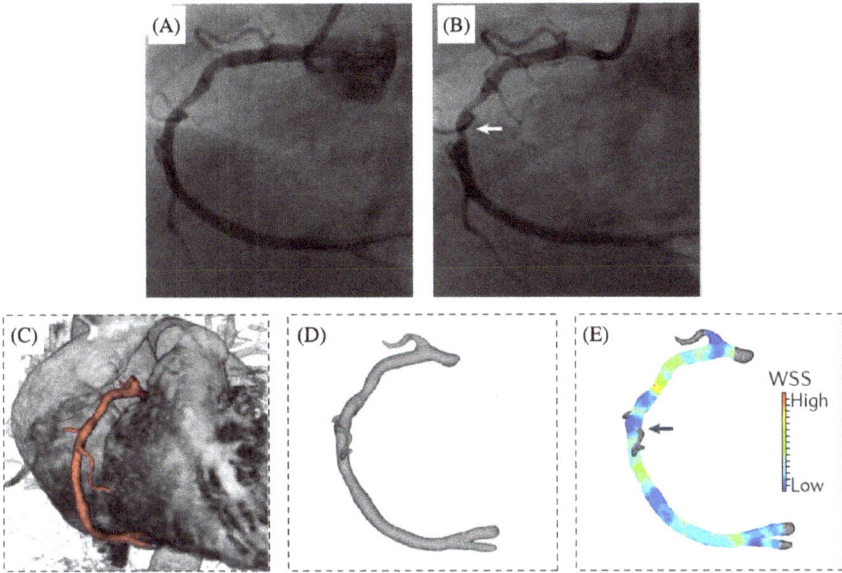

Figure 5.2. WSS calculations. (A) Baseline invasive coronary angiography (ICA) shows an atherosclerotic plaque at the right coronary artery. (B) Repeat coronary angiography performed 4 years later for stable angina shows plaque progression with an increase in lumen narrowing (arrow). (C) 3D volume rendering CT angiography of right coronary artery. (D) 3D reconstruction of coronary geometry based on 3D volume rendering CT images. E: Computational fluid dynamic simulation shows a region of low WSS that is consistent with the plaque progression (arrow). Reprinted with permission from Brown *et al.*[9]

cycle. High OSI refers to flow reversal and varying OSI over a cardiac cycle.

- **RRT**: A metric of species transport. It refers to the duration that a particle remains in a particular subregion with low RRT stimulating thrombus formation and high RRT seen in separated, recirculating flow.

These hemodynamic parameters are possible indicators for atherosclerotic plaque prone sites.[46–49] Of these parameters, low WSS or OSI is a well-studied mechanical stimulus that promotes the inflammatory process by inducing an oxidative response in endothelial vascular cells.[50,51] This has led to the increasing applications of CFD in the investigation of pathogenesis of CAD, in particular, the identification and detection of high-risk plaques.

5.3.1 Coronary CT Angiography-generated Coronary Artery Models

Before performing CFD simulations, an essential step is to acquire high-resolution CCTA images so that an accurate geometry of the coronary artery tree including coronary plaques can be reconstructed. The diameter of normal coronary artery is between 3 and 5 mm in the main segments, and about 1 mm in the distal segments. Detection and quantification of coronary artery stenosis requires coronary CT imaging to be able to distinguish a minimal 20% change in the diameter. To achieve this goal, CT scanners need to provide a spatial resolution with isotropic resolution of at least 0.5 mm in all three dimensions for visualization of the main coronary vessels and of smaller branches. Thus, in-plane and through-plane resolution well below 1.0 mm are required to accurately assess the main coronary segments, including lumen narrowing and plaques. Currently, isotropic volume data can be obtained with latest multislice CT (>64-slice) scanners resulting in 0.35 × 0.35 × 0.35 mm^3, therefore allowing excellent visualization of coronary anatomy and plaque with high diagnostic accuracy (Fig. 5.3).[52–55] High-definition CT scanner with substantially improved in-plane spatial resolution of 0.23 mm has been shown to further improve diagnostic value of CCTA in CAD when compared to standard 64-slice CT scanners, in particular, showing advantages in reducing beam hardening and blooming artifacts due to heavy calcification in coronary plaques.[56]

5.3.2 Wall Shear Stress in Relation to Atherosclerotic Plaque Formation

Since flow in the left coronary artery is more complex than the right side due to branching vessels arising from the left coronary artery, the focus is placed on the hemodynamic parameters in relation to plaque development in the left coronary artery.

Of these hemodynamic parameters, WSS has been shown to be more sensitive than others in prediction of plaque locations and determination

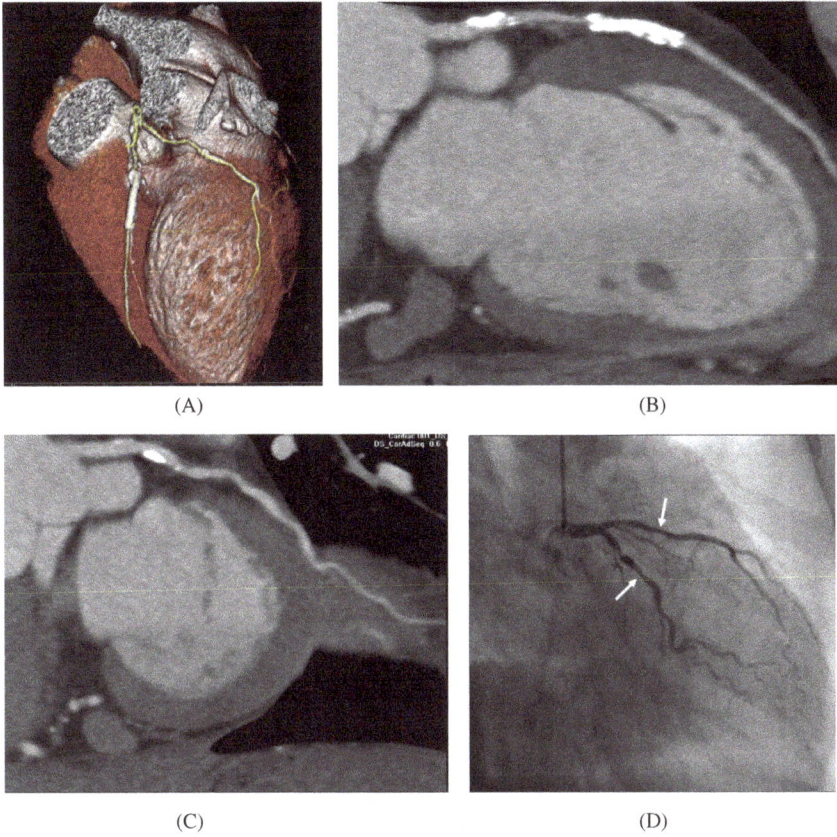

(A)   (B)

(C)   (D)

Figure 5.3.   CCTA in the visualization of coronary artery plaques in a 58-year-old man. (A) 3D volume rendering show multiple plaques in LAD and LCx. (B) and (C) Curved planar reformatted images show calcified plaques in the LAD and LCx branches with significant lumen stenosis. This is confirmed by ICA (arrows in D). Coronary stent is noticed at the LAD as shown in Fig 5.3(A).

of atherosclerotic changes in the coronary artery. An early study based on five patients (three with atherosclerotic plaques and two with normal left coronary arteries) demonstrated the feasibility of CFD simulations in 16-slice CCTA-generated models. WSS increased in the atherosclerotic coronary arteries, while in contrast, the WSS remained low in normal coronary arteries.[57] Later reports based on modern CT scanners further confirmed these findings.

Rikhtegar *et al.* compared average WSS with the other three parameters including OSI, RRT and average wall shear stress gradient (AWSSG) in 30 patient-specific geometrics of the left coronary artery which were acquired with dual-source CT angiographic images.[58] A total of 96 plaques were found to be present at different segments of left coronary artery, with average WSS having the highest sensitivity in predicting plaque locations when compared to other parameters (86 ± 25%, 65 ± 37%, 67 ± 32% and 48 ± 38% corresponding to average WSS, AWSSG, OSI and RRT, respectively) ($p < 0.05$). OSI had higher sensitivity than AWSSG and RRT. RRT has higher positive predictive value (PPV) than average WSS (49 ± 39% vs 31 ± 20%) ($p < 0.05$). The authors concluded that although low WSS represents a prerequisite for plaque formation and atherosclerosis, time-dependent changes of WSS should be considered since low shear stress alone is insufficient to induce plaque formation. This leads to the increasing use of TAWSS in the hemodynamic study of coronary atherosclerotic changes.

Low TAWSS, high OSI and high RRT values were reported to indicate the region of developing atherosclerosis in the left coronary artery.[59] Low WSS has been shown to be closely associated with early plaque or atherosclerotic development.[17,19–24] Currently, there is no consensus about the cut-off values to determine WSS ranges in terms of low, intermediate and high WSS. In general, low WSS is defined as <10 dynes/cm;[2,22,24,60–62] however, intermediate and high WSS are not clearly defined. It is generally agreed that low WSS contributes to initiating atherosclerosis and plaque progression.[63] Despite the reports by some researchers about the relationship between low WSS and development of high-risk plaque,[64,65] most of the studies supported the role for high WSS in the development of high-risk or vulnerable plaque because of direct correlation between focally elevated WSS and the plaque rupture site.[66] This emphasizes the importance of studying WSS changes in relation to the development of high-risk plaque.

5.3.3 WSS Changes and High-risk Plaque

The correlation between high WSS and high-risk or vulnerable plaque has been widely studied, with evidence showing that high WSS is most commonly observed in coronary arteries with large plaque consisting of necrotic core or positive arterial remodeling.

Significant correlation has been reported between high WSS and plaque burden (>40%) in larger plaques.[34,60] Hetterich et al. investigated the relationship between WSS and plaque features based on CFD analysis of CCTA-generated models from seven patients with suspected CAD. Their results showed that increased wall thickness and higher amount of fibrofatty tissue were noted in the locations where coronary artery was exposed to low WSS. The lowest wall thickness was found in the area of high WSS when compared to that with low WSS region (mean wall thickness 0.38 ± 0.32 mm vs 0.43 ± 0.34 mm, $p < 0.001$).[67] Han and colleagues reported similar findings in their recent study comprising 100 patients. High WSS was found to be independently associated with coronary plaque features, with high WSS having 2.5-fold increased odds of positive remodeling and low-attenuation plaque. However, their study concluded that WSS was not an independent predictor of coronary ischemia because there was no direct correlation between high WSS and coronary lesion ischemia.[68]

A recent study by Park et al. has analyzed hemodynamic changes in patient-specific models from 80 patients with plaques located at the left coronary artery tree.[69] Higher WSS (>40 dynes/cm^2) was observed at stenotic coronary segments (diameter stenosis was $52.3 \pm 14.4\%$) when compared with non-stenotic segments. Their findings are in line with other studies demonstrating the association of higher WSS with higher probability of plaque features, with low-attenuation plaque and napkin-ring sign significantly more prevalent in the highest WSS areas (>111.9 dynes/cm^2) when compared to the lowest or middle WSS regions ($p < 0.05$). Their study further confirms the limited role of luminal narrowing by CCTA or invasive angiography in assessing plaque vulnerability, while CFD analysis of hemodynamic changes to the coronary arteries, in particular the WSS changes, offer more valuable information about plaque vulnerability.[70, 71]

Most of the current studies investigating the relationship between WSS changes and advanced atherosclerotic plaques and location of plaque rupture are mainly based on IVUS or optical coherence tomography (OCT)-generated models for CFD simulations. These two imaging techniques have superior spatial resolution, thus providing excellent intravascular views of coronary plaque composition, allowing assessment of plaque characteristics in relation to hemodynamic changes.[72] Due to the invasive nature of these imaging modalities, CCTA-derived CFD simulations are showing great promise, although more studies based on large sample size are needed.

5.3.4 Hemodynamics and Coronary Bifurcation Angle

The correlation between left coronary bifurcation (angle between LAD and LCx) and CAD has been widely studied, with results showing that wide angulation is associated with CAD.[73–77] A bifurcation angle of 80° is commonly used as a cut-off value to determine the presence of CAD, as confirmed by previous studies investigating the natural distribution of coronary bifurcation angles.[74,75] Our experience of analyzing the association between left coronary bifurcation angle and CAD in terms of intraluminal changes caused by coronary plaques are consistent with these findings.[76,77] Irregular intraluminal coronary changes as observed on virtual intravascular endoscopy are seen in more than 50% of patients with bifurcation angle of more than 80°, and in more than 90% of cases with mixed plaques.

Recent studies from our group further confirm the association between left coronary bifurcation and CAD.[78,79] Of 50 patients with suspected CAD undergoing coronary CT angiography, coronary plaques were detected at one or more coronary arteries in 25 patients, while in the remaining 25 patients, as a control group, no plaque was found. The mean bifurcation angle was measured 83.9° ± 17.5° (range, 45°, 112°) in patients with CAD having coronary plaques; in contrast, the mean bifurcation angle was 62.5° ± 15.4° (range, 36°, 89°) in patients with normal coronary artery, showing significant difference ($p < 0.001$) (Figs. 5.4 and 5.5).[78] In a retrospective study comprising 196 patients, the left bifurcation angle was investigated to determine its relationship with common risk factors for developing CAD, such as body mass index (BMI), gender, hypertension, diabetes, cholesterol levels, smoking and family history.[79] Results showed significant associations of BMI and gender with bifurcation angle. Males were found to have at least

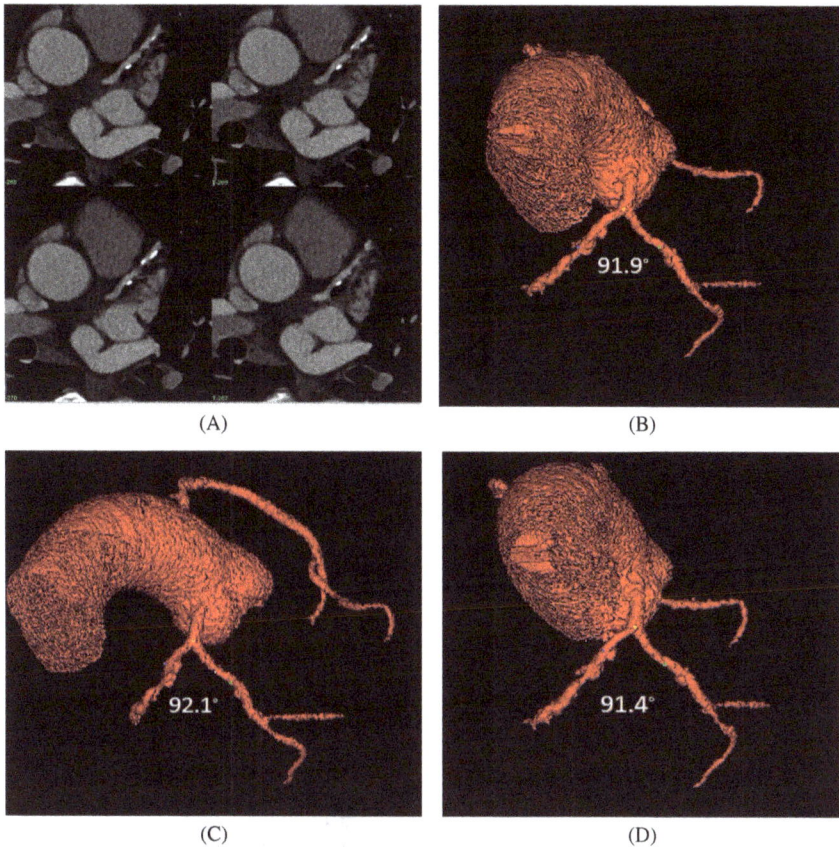

(A)   (B)

(C)   (D)

Figure 5.4. Association between wide angulation and CAD in a 52-year-old man with CAD. (A) 2D axial images show multiple calcified plaques at the LAD artery. (B)–(D) Left coronary bifurcation angle between LAD and LCx was measured at three different positions with the mean angulation of 91.8° indicating significant coronary stenosis. Reprinted with permission under the open access from Sun and Lee.[78]

2.07-fold greater risk of having a >80° bifurcation angle and developing CAD than females ($p = 0.003$), and patients with large BMI (>25 kg/ m^2) were 2.54-fold more likely to have a >80° bifurcation angle than patients with a normal BMI ($p = 0.001$).[79] Despite its retrospective nature, this study adds valuable information to the current literature by clarifying the direct association between left bifurcation angle and some risk factors, although only low to intermediate risk patients were included in the study with most of the cases being normal. These findings were confirmed by a recent single-center study comprising 313 patients who underwent CCTA with analysis of the bifurcation angle in relation to patients with CAD (significant vs non-significant stenosis).[80] Findings of this study showed significant correlation between left coronary bifurcation angle and coronary atherosclerotic disease, with the mean angle being 87.3°, 81.32° and 75.5° ($p < 0.001$), corresponding to the group of patients with significant coronary stenosis (≥50%), CAD without significant stenosis and unremarkable CCTA with calcium score of zero. The authors further determined the significant correlation between these risk factors, including male gender, diabetes mellitus, obesity, hypertension and BMI, and left coronary bifurcation angle ($p < 0.05$). Further, the authors, for the first time, demonstrated the feasibility of using axial images to visualize and measure left coronary bifurcation angle (Fig. 5.6).

It is well known that diagnostic value of CCTA is affected by heavy or severely calcified plaques, with low specificity and PPV (less than 50%) due to blooming artifacts from the calcified plaques.[81–84] The diagnostic value of left coronary bifurcation angle has been demonstrated in the assessment of calcified plaques with improved diagnostic performance.[85,86] In a recent study, a direction comparison was performed in 53 patients with calcified plaques detected on CCTA. Diagnostic value of CCTA using bifurcation angle was compared with that from the conventional coronary lumen assessment with ICA as the reference method. The specificity and PPV of CCTA by bifurcation angle showed significant improvement over the coronary lumen assessment, with corresponding values being 79% (95% CI 59%, 92%) and 81% (95% CI 62%, 92%) for bifurcation angle-based diagnosis, and 33% (95% CI 21%, 47%) and 43% (95% CI 31%, 56%) for minimal lumen diameter-based diagnosis, respectively, while sensitivity and negative predictive value remained unchanged (100% for both approaches).[86]

The role of bifurcation angle in relation to CAD or plaque formation was further confirmed by studies based on CCTA-derived CFD analysis. Idealized coronary models with various angles to simulate left coronary bifurcation have shown low WSS in the models with wide angulations.[4,87]

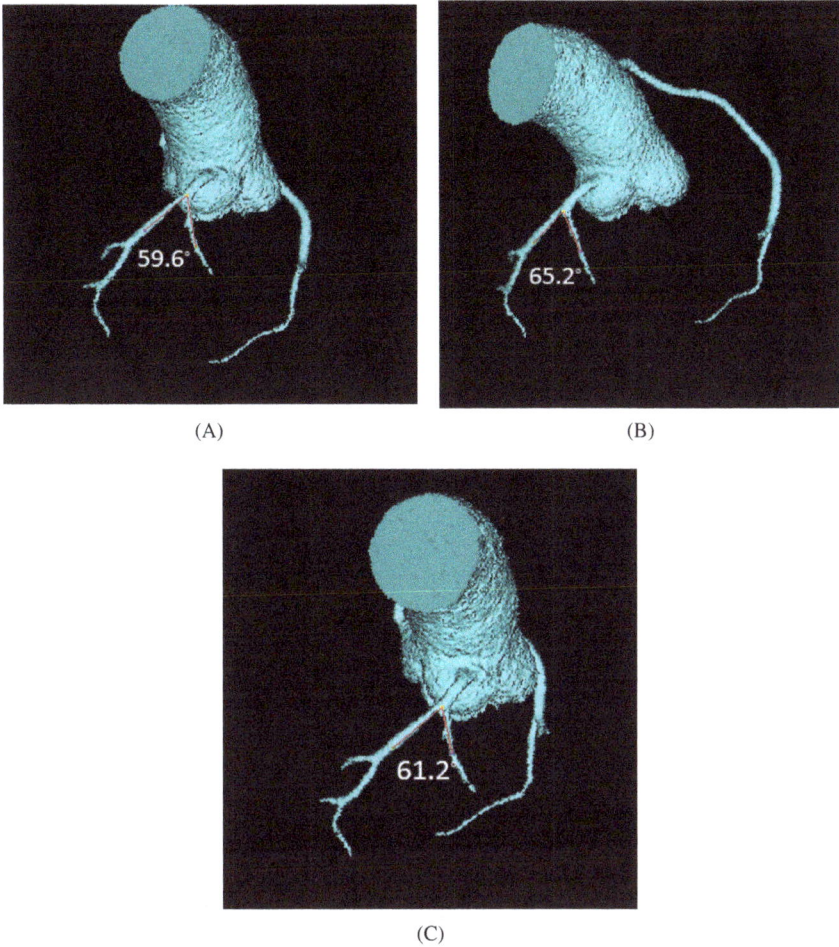

(A)   (B)

(C)

Figure 5.5.   Association between narrow angulation and normal coronary artery in a 55-year-old female. (A)–(C) Left coronary bifurcation angle between LAD and LCx was measured at three different positions with the mean angle of 62° indicating no significant coronary disease. Reprinted with permission under the open access from Sun and Lee.[78]

Similar findings were noticed in CFD simulations using realistic models based on CCTA-generated models with hemodynamic analysis more accurate than coronary lumen assessment for determination of significant stenosis. Chaichana and Sun analyzed 11 patients with calcified plaques at the left coronary artery and compared CFD simulations based on

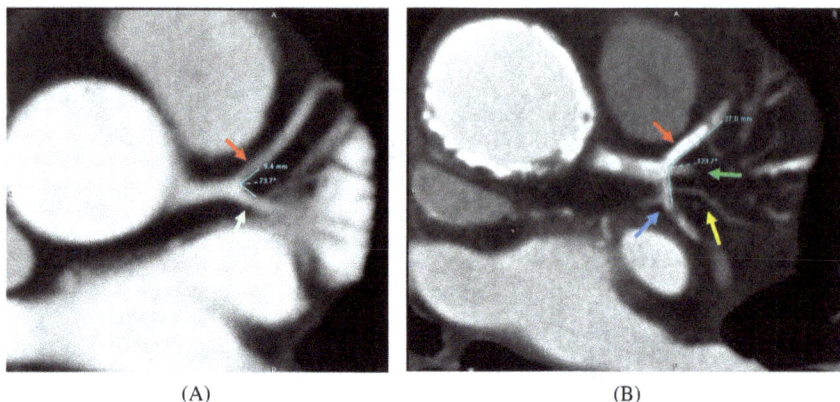

(A)   (B)

Figure 5.6.   2D axial images measuring left coronary bifurcation angle. (A) Normal findings of the LAD coronary artery and LCx with zero calcium score, and the angle between LAD and LCx of 73.7°. (B) Significant stenosis of the LAD and LCx due to calcified plaques, with calcium score of 690 at LAD and total calcium score of 3,775. The bifurcation angle between LAD and LCx was measured 123.7°. The ramus intermedius (green arrow) and obtuse marginal branch 1 (yellow arrow) are also clearly displayed in the axial image. Reprinted with permission under the open access from Juan *et al.*[80].

CCTA-generated models with coronary lumen stenosis.[88] Of these patients, 15 significant stenotic lesions were detected by CCTA at the left coronary artery; however, only three of them were confirmed to be significant stenosis (>50%) on ICA. WSS was found to increase in the left coronary artery models with angulation >80°, but remained little or no change in the narrow angulated models. Flow velocity increased at the post-stenotic regions as shown in Figs. 5.7 and 5.8.[88]

Plaques located at the left bifurcation region also have a significant impact on the hemodynamic flow to the coronary artery according to our experience of CFD coronary simulations based on idealized and realistic models.[89–91] With different types of plaques simulated at the LAD and LCx arteries, we analyzed and characterized hemodynamic effects associated with each type of plaque. When the left main stem and other two left coronary artery branches were involved with plaques, velocity and wall pressure gradient were found to be the highest, while significant changes of velocity, WSS and pressure gradient were noted with plaques located at

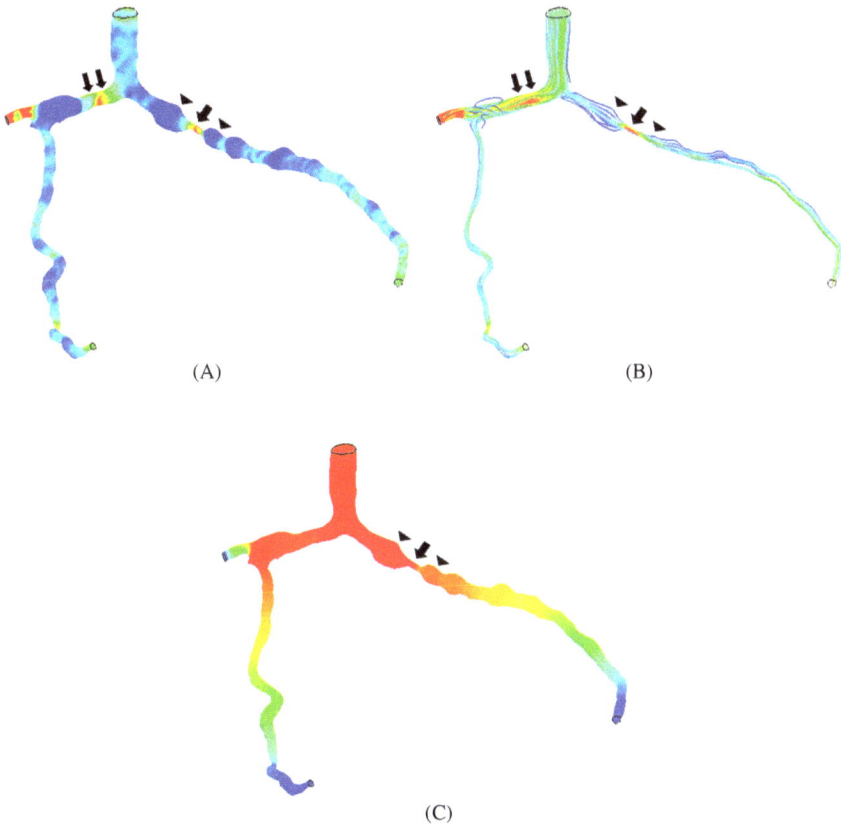

(A)   (B)

(C)

Figure 5.7. Relationship between wide bifurcation angle and hemodynamic changes by CFD analysis. Left coronary bifurcation angle between LAD and LCx was measured 108° with significant stenosis of LAD and LCx on coronary CT angiography but with LCx >50% stenosis confirmed on ICA in a 65-year-old man. WSS and flow velocity were increased, in particular at the LCx (A and B, with arrow in B showing significant stenosis in LCx), with decreased wall pressure at the stenotic lesion (arrow in C).

the LCx ($p < 0.001$).[90] Similar findings were reported in patient-specific CFD simulations in another study from our group. Left coronary artery models were generated from CCTA in 22 patients with CAD with coronary plaques present in at least one of the left coronary branches with stenosis ranging from 25% to 70%. WSS was increased significantly at the left coronary artery with significant stenosis (>70%), with WSS

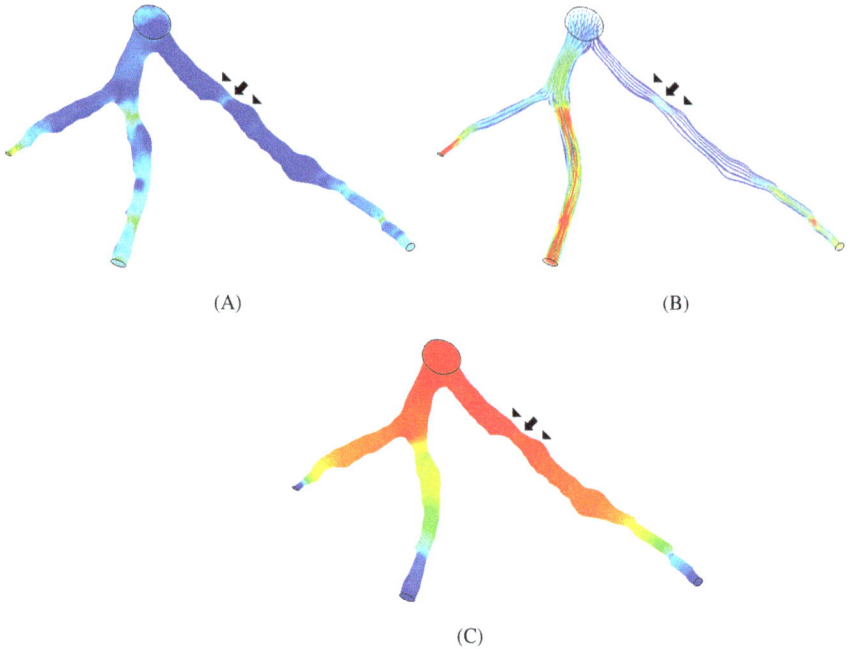

(A)   (B)

(C)

Figure 5.8. Relationship between narrow bifurcation angle and hemodynamic changes by CFD analysis. Left coronary bifurcation angle between LAD and LCx was measured 71° with significant stenosis of LCx on coronary CT angiography but showing less than 50% stenosis on ICA in a 54-year-old man. WSS, flow velocity and wall pressure did not show significant change (A-C). Arrows refer to the area of non-significant stenotic regions in LCx.

ranging from 2.5 to 3.5 Pa, while in the coronary artery with intermediate stenosis (<50%), the corresponding WSS values were either <1 Pa or between 1 and 2.5 Pa.[91] These findings are consistent with other reports, confirming the association between geometric vasculature in the coronary artery and development of CAD.[92,93] CCTA-derived CFD simulations showed direct correlation between left coronary bifurcation angle and significant coronary stenosis in the diagnostic assessment of calcified plaques, with significant improvement in specificity and PPV when diagnosis was based on bifurcation angle in comparison with the conventional coronary lumen assessment (specificity and PPV were 78.6% and 84.2%, 52% and 49%) respectively.[93]

5.4 Summary and Conclusion

CCTA represents the latest technological development in cardiac imaging, with excellent spatial and temporal resolution, allowing visualization and assessment of coronary artery anatomy as well as characterization of coronary plaques with high diagnostic value. Furthermore, CCTA allows generation of patient-specific coronary models; therefore, CCTA-derived CFD simulations have been increasingly used for analysis of hemodynamic changes to determine the location of coronary plaque formation and identify high-risk plaques. Studies using idealized and realistic coronary models have demonstrated the feasibility of CFD simulations, with results offering insight into hemodynamic changes to the coronary artery in relation to different types of plaques. Further clarification of relationship between coronary plaques and hemodynamic significant stenosis with myocardial ischemic changes will be discussed in the next chapter, CCTA-derived fractional flow reserve, which is a hot topic, but still debatable in terms of its clinical application in the current practice.

References

1. Shaaban AM, Duerinckx AJ. (2000) Wall shear stress and early atherosclerosis: a review. *AJR Am J Roentgenol* **174**: 1657–1665.
2. Cunningham KS, Gotlieb AI. (2005) The role of shear stress in the pathogenesis of atherosclerosis. *Lab Invest* **85**: 9–23.
3. Davies PF, Polacek DC, Shi C, Helmke BP. (2002) The convergence of haemodynamics, genomics, and endothelial structure in studies of the focal origin of atherosclerosis. *Biorheology* **39**: 299–306.
4. Chaichana T, Sun Z, Jewkes J. (2011) Computation of hemodynamics in the left coronary artery with variable angulations. *J Biomech* **44**: 1869–1878.
5. Zarins CK, Giddens DP, Bharadvaj BK, Sottiuria VS, Mabon RF, Glagov S. (1983) Carotid bifurcation atherosclerosis. Quantitative correlation of plaque localization with flow velocity profiles and wall shear stress. *Circ Res* **53**: 502–514.
6. Ku D N, Giddens DP, Zarins CK, Glagov S. (1985) Pulsatile flow and atherosclerosis in the human carotid bifurcation. Positive correlation between plaque location and low oscillating shear stress. *Arteriosclerosis* **5**: 293–302.
7. Chiu JJ, Chien S. (2011) Effects of disturbed flow on vascular endothelium: pathophysiological basis and clinical perspectives. *Physiol Rev* **91**: 327–387.
8. Taylor CA, Fonte TA, Min JK. (2013) Computational fluid dynamics applied to cardiac computed tomography for noninvasive quantification of fractional flow reserve: scientific basis. *J Am Coll Cardiol* **61**: 2233–2241.

9. Brown AJ, Teng Z, Evans PC *et al.* (2016) Role of biomechanical forces in the natural history of coronary atherosclerosis. *Nat Rev Cardiol* **13**: 210–220.

10. Lee BK, Kwon HM, Hong BK *et al.* (2001) Hemodynamic effects on atherosclerosis-prone coronary artery: wall shear stress/rate distribution and impedance phase angle in coronary and aortic circulation. *Yonsei Med J* **42**: 375–383.

11. Wong KK, Sun Z, Tu J, Worthley SG, Mazumdar J, Abbott D. (2012) Medical image diagnostics based on computer-aided flow analysis using magnetic resonance images. *Comput Med Imaging Graph* **36**: 527–541.

12. Coskun AU, Yeghiazarians Y, Kinlay S *et al.* (2003) Reproducibility of coronary lumen, plaque, and vessel wall reconstruction and of endothelial shear stress measurements *in vivo* in humans. *Catheter Cardiovasc Interv* **60**: 67–78.

13. Stone PH, Coskun AU, Yeghiazarians Y *et al.* (2003) Prediction of sites of coronary atherosclerosis progression: in vivo profiling of endothelial shear stress, lumen, and outer vessel wall characteristics to predict vascular behavior. *Curr Opin Cardiol* **18**: 458–470.

14. Stone PH, Coskun AU, Kinlay S *et al.* (2007) Regions of low endothelial shear stress are the sites where coronary plaque progresses and vascular remodelling occurs in humans: an in vivo serial study. *Eur Heart J* **28**: 705–710.

15. Lee BK. (2011) Computational fluid dynamics in cardiovascular disease. *Korean Circ J* **41**: 423–430.

16. Lee BK, Kwon HM, Kim DS *et al.* (1998) Computed numerical analysis of the biomechanical effects on coronary atherogenesis using human hemodynamic and dimensional variables. *Yonsei Med J* **39**: 166–174.

17. Wahle A, Lopez JJ, Olszewski ME *et al.* (2008) Plaque development, vessel curvature, and wall shear stress in coronary arteries assessed by x-ray angiography and intravascular ultrasound. *Med Image Anal* **10**: 615–631.

18. van der Giessen AG, Schaap M, Gijsen FJ *et al.* (2009) 3D fusion of intravascular ultrasound and coronary computed tomography for in-vivo wall shear stress analysis: a feasibility study. *Int J Cardiovasc Imaging* **26**: 781–796.

19. LaDisa JF, Bowers M, Harmann L *et al.* (2010) Time-efficient patient-specific quantification of regional carotid artery fluid dynamics and spatial correlation with plaque burden. *Med Phys* **37**: 784–792.

20. Gijsen FJH, Schuurbiers JCH, van de Giessen AG, Schaap M, van der Steen AF, Wentzel JJ. (2014) 3D reconstruction techniques of human coronary bifurcations for shear stress computations. *J Biomech* **47**: 39–43.

21. Stone PH, Coskun AU, Kinlay S *et al.* (2003) Effect of endothelial shear stress on the progression of coronary artery disease, vascular remodeling, and in-stent restenosis in humans: in vivo 6-month follow-up study. *Circulation* **108**: 438–444.

22. Stone PH, Saito S, Takahashi S *et al.* (2012) Prediction of progression of coronary artery disease and clinical outcomes using vascular profiling of endothelial shear stress and arterial plaque characteristics: the PREDICTION study. *Circulation* **126**: 172–181.

23. Corban MT, Eshtehardi P, Suo J *et al.* (2014) Combination of plaque burden, wall shear stress, and plaque phenotype has incremental value for prediction of coronary atherosclerotic plaque progression and vulnerability. *Atherosclerosis* **232**: 271–276.

24. Samady H, Eshtehardi P, McDaniel MC *et al.* (2011) Coronary artery wall shear stress is associated with progression and transformation of atherosclerotic plaque and arterial remodeling in patients with coronary artery disease. *Circulation* **124**: 779–788.

25. Schiemann M, Bakhtiary F, Hietschold V *et al.* (2006) MR-based coronary artery blood velocity measurements in patients without coronary artery disease. *Eur Radiol* **16**: 1124–1130.

26. Nichols W, O'Rourke M. (2005) *McDonald's Blood Flow in Arteries.* London: Hodder Arnold.

27. Timmins LH, Molony DS, Eshtehardi P *et al.* (2015) Focal association between wall shear stress and clinical coronary artery disease progression. *Ann. Biomed. Eng* **43**: 94–106.

28. Pedrigi RM, Mehta VV, Bovens SM *et al.* (2016) Influence of shear stress magnitude and direction on atherosclerotic plaque composition. *R Soc Open Sci* **3**: 160558.

29. He X, Ku ND. (1996) Pulsatile flow in the human left coronary artery bifurcation: average conditions. *J Biomech Eng* **118**: 74–82.

30. Katritsis DG, Theodorakakos A, Pantos I *et al.* (2010) Vortex formation and recirculation zones in left anterior descending artery stenosis: Computational fluid dynamics analysis. *Phys Med Biol* **55**: 1395–1411.

31. Katritsis D, Kaiktsis L, Chaniotis A, Pantos J, Efstathopoulos F, Marmarelis V. (2007) Wall shear stress: theoretical considerations and methods of measurement. *Prog Cardiovasc Dis* **49**: 307–329.

32. Katritsis DG, Pantos I, Efstathopoulos F. (2007) Hemodynamic factors and atheromatic plaque rupture in the coronary arteries: from vulnerable plaque to vulnerable coronary segment. *Coron Artery Dis* **18**: 229–237.

33. Boutsianis E, Dave H, Frauenfelder T *et al.* (2004) Computational simulation of intracoronary flow based on real coronary geometry. *Eur J Cardiothorac Surg* **26**: 248–256.

34. Wellnhofer E, Goubergrits L, Kertzscher U, Affeld K. (2006) In-vivo coronary flow profiling based on biplane angiograms: influence of geometric simplifications on three-dimensional reconstruction and wall shear stress calculation. *Biomed Eng Online* **5**: 39.

35. Dong J, Sun Z, Inthavong K, Tu J. (2015) Fluid-structure interaction analysis of the left coronary artery with variable angulations. *Comput Med Biomech Biomed Eng* **18**: 1500–1508.

36. Siauw WL, Ng EYK, Mazumdar J. (2000) Unsteady stenosis flow prediction: a comparative study of non-Newtonian models with operator splitting scheme. *Med Eng Phys* **22**: 265–277.

37. Lantz J, Renner J, Karlsson M. (2011) Wall shear stress in a subject specific human aora-influence of fluid-structure interactions. Int J Appl Mech **3**: 759–778.
38. Hei M, Hazel AL. (2011) Fluid-structure interaction in internal physiological flows. Annu Rev Fluid Mech **43**: 141–162.
39. Vigmostad SC, Udaykumar HS, Lu J, Chandran KB. (2010) Fluid-structure interaction methods in biological flows with special emphasis on heart valve dynamics. Int J Numer Methods Biomed Eng **26**: 435–470.
40. Tezduyar TE, Takizawa K, Brummer T, Chen PR. (2011) Space-time fluid-structure interaction modeling of patient-specific cerebral aneurysms. Int J Numer Methods Biomed Eng **27**: 1665–1710.
41. Torii R, Oshima M, Kobayashi T, Takagi K, Tezduyar TE. (2009) Fluid-structure interaction modeling of blood flow and cerebral aneurysm: significance of artery and aneurysm shapes. Comput Methods Appl Mech Eng **198**: 3613–3621.
42. Qiao A, Guo X, Wu S, Zeng Y, Xu X. (2004) Numerical study of nonlinear pulsatile flow in s-shaped curved arteries. Med Eng Phys **26**: 545–552.
43. Liu Q, Mirc D, Fu BM. (2008) Mechanical mechanisms of thrombosis in intact bent microvessels of rat mesentery. J Biomech **41**: 2726–2734.
44. Xie X, Wang Y, Zhu H, Zhou J. (2014) Computation of hemodynamics in tortuous left coronary artery: a morphological parametric study. J Biomech Eng **136**: 101006.
45. Davies PF. (1995) Flow-mediated endothelial mechanotransduction. Physiol Rev **75**: 519–560.
46. Buchanan Jr JR, Kleinstreuer C, Truskey GA, Lei M. (1999) Relation between non-uniform hemodynamics and sites of altered permeability and lesion growth at the rabbit aorto-celiac junction. Atherosclerosis **143**: 27–40.
47. Chatzizisis YS, Jonas M, Coskun AU et al. (2008) Prediction of the localization of high risk coronary atherosclerotic plaques on the basis of low endothelial shear stress: an intravascular ultrasound and histopathology natural history study. Circulation **117**: 993–1002.
48. Chatzizisis YS, Coskun AU, Jonas M, Edelman ER, Feldman CL, Stone PH. (2007) Role of endothelial shear stress in the natural history of coronary atherosclerosis and vascular remodeling: molecular, cellular, and vascular behavior. J Am Coll Cardiol **49**: 2379–2393.
49. Himburg HA, Grzybowski DM, Hazel AL, LaMack JA, Li XM, Friedman MH. (2004) Spatial comparison between wall shear stress measures and porcine arterial endothelial permeability. Am J Physiol Heart Circ Physiol **286**: H1916–H1922.
50. Lehoux S, Castier Y, Tedgui A. (2006) Molecular mechanisms of the vascular responses to haemodynamic forces. J Intern Med **259**: 381–392.
51. Lehoux S. (2006) Redox signalling in vascular responses to shear and stretch. Cardiovasc Res **71**: 269–279.
52. Sun Z, Choo GH, Ng KH. (2012) Coronary CT angiography: current status and continuing challenges. Br J Radiol **85**: 495–510.

53. Sun Z. (2012) Cardiac CT imaging: current status and future directions. *Quant Imaging Med Surg* **2**: 98–105.

54. Sun Z. (2013) Cardiac imaging in the diagnosis of coronary artery disease: a comprehensive review of various imaging modalities. *Curr Med Imaging Rev* **9**: 167–169.

55. Machida H, Tanaka I, Fukui R *et al.* (2015) Current and novel imaging techniques in coronary CT. *Radiographics* **35**: 991–1010.

56. Pontone G, Bertella E, Mushtaq S *et al.* (2014) Coronary artery disease: diagnostic accuracy of CT coronary angiography — a comparison of high and standard spatial resolution scanning. *Radiology* **271**: 688–694.

57. Frauenfelder T, Boutsianis E, Schertler T *et al.* (2007) *In vivo* flow simulation in coronary arteries based on computed tomography datasets: feasibility and initial results. *Eur Radiol* **17**: 1291–1300.

58. Rikhtegar F, Knight JA, Olgac U *et al.* (2012) Choosing the optimal wall shear parameter for the prediction of plaque location — a patient-specific computational study in human left coronary arteries. *Atherosclerosis* **221**: 432–437.

59. Pinto SIS, Campos JBLM. (2016) Numerical study of wall shear stress-based descriptors in the human left coronary artery. *Comput Methods Biomech Biomed Engin* **19**: 1443–1455.

60. Eshtehardi P, McDaniel MC, Suo J *et al.* (2012) Association of coronary wall shear stress with atherosclerotic plaque burden, composition, and distribution in patients with coronary artery disease. *J Am Heart Assoc* **1**: e002543.

61. Vergallo R, Papafaklis MI, Yonetsu T *et al.* (2014) Endothelial shear stress and coronary plaque characteristics in humans: combined frequency-domain optical coherence tomography and computational fluid dynamics study. *Circ Cardiovasc Imaging* **7**: 905–911.

62. Eshtehardi P, Brown AJ, Bhargava A *et al.* (2017) High wall shear stress and high-risk plaque: an emerging concept. *Int J Cardiovasc Imaging* **33**: 1089–1099.

63. Wentzel JJ, Chatzizisis YS, Gijsen FJ, Giannoglou GD, Feldman CL, Stone PH. (2012) Endothelial shear stress in the evolution of coronary atherosclerotic plaque and vascular remodelling: current understanding and remaining questions. *Cardiovasc Res* **96**: 234–243.

64. Zaromytidou M, Siasos G, Coskun AU *et al.* (2016) Intravascular hemodynamics and coronary artery disease: new insights and clinical implications. *Hellenic J Cardiol* **57**: 389–400.

65. Fukumoto Y, Hiro T, Fujii T *et al.* (2008) Localized elevation of shear stress is related to coronary plaque rupture: a 3-dimensional intravascular ultrasound study with *in-vivo* color mapping of shear stress distribution. *J Am Coll Cardiol* **51**: 645–650.

66. Kwak BR, Back M, Bochaton-Piallat ML *et al.* (2014) Biomechanical factors in atherosclerosis: mechanisms and clinical implications. *Eur Heart J* **35**: 3013–3020.

67. Hetterich H, Jaber A, Gehring M *et al.* (2015) Coronary computed tomography angiography based assessment of endothelial shear stress and its association with atherosclerotic plaque distribution *in vivo. PLOS One* **10**: e0115408.

68. Han D, Starikov A, o Hartaigh B *et al.* (2016) Relationship between endothelial wall shear stress and high-risk atherosclerotic plaque characteristics for identification of coronary lesions that cause ischemia: a direct comparison with fractional flow reserve. *J Am Heart Assoc* **5**: e004186.

69. Park JB, Choi G, Chun EJ *et al.* (2016) Computational fluid dynamic measures of wall shear stress are related to coronary lesion characteristics. *Heart* **102**(20): 1655–1661.

70. Fishbein MC, Siegel RJ. (1996) How big are coronary atherosclerotic plaques that rupture? *Circulation* **94**: 2662–2666.

71. Chan KH, Ng MKC. (2013) Is there a role for coronary angiography in the early detection of the vulnerable plaque? *Int J Cardiol* **164**: 262–266.

72. Gijsen F, van der Giessen A, van der Steen A, Wentzel J. (2013) Shear stress and advanced atherosclerosis in human coronary arteries. *J Biomech* **46**: 240–247.

73. Rodriguez-Granillo GA, Garcia-Garcia HM, Wentzel J *et al.* (2006) Plaque composition and its relationship with acknowledged shear stress patterns in coronary arteries. *J Am Coll Cardiol* **47**(4): 884–885.

74. Reig J, Petit M. (2004) Main trunk of the left coronary artery: anatomic study of the parameters of clinical interest. *Clin Anat* **17**(1): 6–13.

75. Pflederer T, Ludwig J, Ropers D, Daniel WG, Achenbach S. (2006) Measurement of coronary artery bifurcation angles by multidetector computed tomography. *Invest Radiol* **41**(11): 793–798.

76. Sun Z, Cao Y. (2011) Multislice CT angiography assessment of left coronary artery: correlation between bifurcation angle and dimensions and development of coronary artery disease. *Eur J Radiol* **79**(2): e90–e95.

77. Sun Z. (2013) Coronary CT angiography in coronary artery disease: correlation between virtual intravascular endoscopic appearances and left bifurcation angulation and coronary plaques. *Biomed Int Res* **2013**: 732059.

78. Sun Z, Lee SY. (2016) Diagnostic value of coronary CT angiography with use of left coronary bifurcaiton angle in coronary artery disease. *Heart Res Open J* **3**: 19–25.

79. Temov K, Sun Z. (2016) Coronary computed tomography angiography investigation of the association between left main coronary artery bifurcation angle and risk factors of coronary artery disease. *Int J Cardiovasc Imaging* **32** (Suppl 1): S129–S137.

80. Juan YH, Tsay PK, Shen WC, Yeh CS, Wen MS, Wan YL. (2017) Comparison of the left main coronary bifurcating angle among patients with normal, non-significantly and significantly stenosed left coronary arteries. *Sci Rep* **7**: 1515.

81. Park MJ, Jung JI, Choi YS *et al.* (2011) Coronary CT angiography in patients with high calcium score: evaluation of plaque characteristics and diagnostic accuracy. *Int J Cardiovasc Imaging* **27**: 43–51.

82. Chen CC, Chen CC, Hsieh IC *et al.* (2011) The effect of calcium score on the diagnostic accuracy of coronary computed tomography angiography. *Int J Cardiovasc Imaging* **27**(Suppl 1): 37–42.

83. Palumbo A, Maffei E, Martini C *et al.* (2009) Coronary calcium score as gatekeeper for 64-slice computed tomography coronary angiography in patients with chest pain: per-segment and per-patient analysis. *Eur Radiol* **19**: 2127–2135.

84. Uehara M, Funabashi N, Takaoka H, Fujimoto Y, Kobayashi Y. (2014) False-positive findings in 320-slice cardiac CT for detection of severe coronary stenosis in comparison with invasive coronary angiography indicate poor prognosis for occurrence of MACE. *Int J Cardiol* **172**: 235–237.

85. Xu L, Sun Z. (2015) Coronary CT angiography evaluation of calcified coronary plaques by measurement of left coronary bifurcation angle. *Int J Cardiol* **182**: 229–231.

86. Sun Z, Xu L, Fan Z. (2016) Coronary CT angiography in calcified coronary plaques: Comparison of diagnostic accuracy between bifurcation angle measurement and coronary lumen assessment for diagnosing significant coronary stenosis. *Int J Cardiol* **203**: 78–86.

87. Chiastra C, Gallo D, Tasso P *et al.* (2017) Healthy and diseased coronary bifurcation geometries influence near-wall and intravascular flow: A computational exploration of the hemodynamic risk. *J Biomech* **58**: 79–88.

88. Sun Z, Chaichana T. (2016) Computational fluid dynamic analysis of calcified coronary plaques: correlation between hemodynamic changes and cardiac image analysis based on left coronary bifurcation angle and lumen assessments. *Interv Cardiol* **8**: 713–719.

89. Chaichana T, Sun Z, Jewkes J. (2012) Investigation of the haemodynamic environment of bifurcation plaques within the left coronary artery in realistic patient models based on CT images. *Australas Phys Eng Sci Med* **35**(2): 231–236.

90. Chaichana T, Sun Z, Jewkes J. (2013) Haemodynamic analysis of the effect of different types of plaqaues in the left coronary artery. *Comput Med Imaging Graph* **37**: 197–206.

91. Chaichana T, Sun Z, Jewkes J. (2013) Hemodynamic impacts of various types of stenosis in the left coronary artery bifurcation: a patient-specific analysis. *Phys Med* **29**(5): 447–452.

92. Zhu H, Ding Z, Piana RN, Gehrig TR, Friedman MH. (2009) Cataloguing the geometry of the human coronary arteries: a potential tool for predicting risk of coronary artery disease. *Int J Cardiol* **135**: 43–52.

93. Sun Z, Chaichana T. (2017) An invesigation of correlation between left coronary bifurcaiton angle and hemodynamic changes in coronary stenosis by coronary computed tomography-derived computational fluid dynamics. *Quant Imaging Med Surg* **7**: 537–548

6 Coronary CT Angiography-Derived Fractional Flow Reserve in Coronary Artery Disease

Table of Contents

Abstract

Although coronary computed tomography angiography (CCTA) has high sensitivity and negative predictive value in the diagnosis of coronary artery disease (CAD), it has low to moderate specificity and positive predictive value. It is a well-known excellent imaging modality for demonstration of anatomical details of coronary artery and visualization of coronary plaques; however, its diagnostic value in identifying hemodynamically significant coronary lesions is relatively poor. This limitation has been addressed by a recently introduced technique, CCTA-derived fractional flow reserve (FFR_{CT}). There is increasing evidence to show that FFR_{CT} correlates well with invasive FFR and demonstrates improved diagnostic performance over CCTA in the detection of ischemic lesions. This chapter provides an overview of the current clinical applications of FFR_{CT} in the diagnosis of significant coronary stenosis. Limitations and challenges of this technique are discussed and highlighted.

Keywords: coronary computed tomography, coronary artery disease, diagnosis, fractional flow reserve, sensitivity, specificity, stenosis.

6.1 Introduction

Coronary computed tomography angiography (CCTA) is one of the most commonly used imaging modalities for diagnostic assessment of coronary artery disease (CAD). CCTA has been shown to have high diagnostic value, in particular, high sensitivity and very high negative predictive value (NPV), which allows it to be widely used as a reliable technique for excluding CAD.[1-8] However, CCTA suffers from one main limitation, which is overestimation of the degree of coronary stenosis, thus leading to increased referral of patients for undergoing downstream testing such as invasive coronary angiography (ICA).[9-11]

The reason for CCTA to perform less well in terms of low positive predictive value (PPV) is due to the difficulty in differentiating coronary stenosis between 50–69% and >70%, most likely because of variable center expertise and inclusion of different patient characteristics.[12-14] Coronary stenosis of >70% is widely accepted as an anatomical threshold to determine significant lumen stenosis. The presence of severe calcification makes interpretation of CCTA images even more difficult due to blooming and beam-hardening artifacts which enlarge plaque volume and compromise accurate visualization and assessment of the coronary lumen stenosis.[15-17] CCTA is mainly used in patients with low to intermediate risk of CAD since patients with high-risk CAD will benefit from ICA for the purpose of revascularization.[18] It has been reported that in patients with high-risk or high-pretest probability of CAD, normal CCTA failed to rule out significant coronary stenosis, indicating that the majority of symptomatic patients still proceed to ICA, despite negative CCTA results.[19] In contrast, CCTA plays an important role in patients with low to intermediate risk of CAD because CCTA findings will directly affect the necessity for additional imaging examinations, and avoid unnecessary ICA in patients with normal CCTA findings.

It is well known that degree of lumen stenosis as assessed on CCTA or ICA is a poor indicator of physiological significance of a stenosis as the visually assessed severity poorly correlates with reduction in myocardial blood flow.[20,21] This is especially apparent in assessing calcified plaques with high false positive rates, leading to low specificity and PPV.[15-17] Therefore, functional assessment of coronary lesions in addition to lumen narrowing is required for optimal diagnosis and management of patients with moderate lumen stenosis. This is achieved with use of fractional flow reserve (FFR), which allows for deciding functional significance of coronary stenosis. FFR can be performed either via invasive approach through coronary angiographic procedure, which is not commonly performed, or through a less invasive method, which is CCTA-derived FFR (FFR_{CT}). In the following sections, an overview of clinical application of invasive FFR is provided, with a focus on the diagnostic value of FFR_{CT} based on the current evidence in the literature.

6.2 Clinical Application of FFR

FFR is the reference method for determining lesion-specific ischemia. It is a lesion-specific index defined as the ratio of maximal coronary pressure distal to a diseased lesion to the proximal maximal aortic pressure during hyperemia. Figure 6.1 is a diagram showing FFR measurement. A shown in the figure, a pressure-sensitive 0.014″ guidewire is positioned distal to a coronary lesion with the aim of determining the physiological or functional significance of a coronary lesion.[22]

There is a linear relationship between coronary flow and pressure with FFR ratio of 1.0 in a normal epicardial coronary artery without any stenosis or obstruction. An FFR of 0.8 indicates that 80% of the normal maximal blood flow is supplied by the diseased coronary artery due to stenosis.

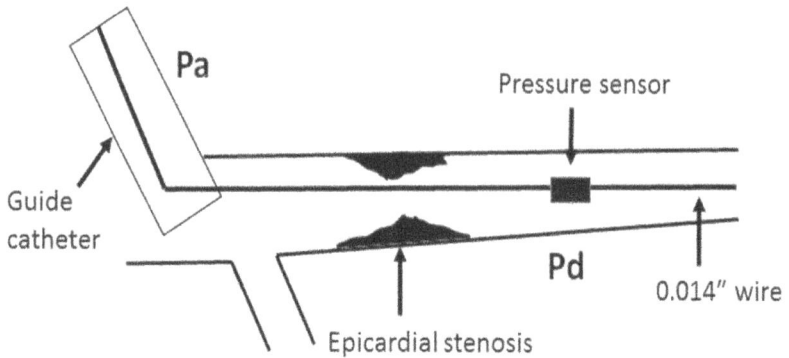

Figure 6.1. Schematic representation of fractional flow reserve measurement during ICA. Pa: proximal (aortic) pressure, Pd: distal coronary pressure. Modified from Corcoran et al.[22]

A clinical cut-off threshold of ≤0.8 is commonly used to define a hemodynamically significant stenosis, while FFR of >0.8 is not considered to induce ischemia.[23]

The clinical value of FFR-guided strategy in patient management has been extensively studied with sufficient evidence showing the beneficial effect of FFR-guided percutaneous coronary intervention (PCI).[24–30] The DEFER (Deferral Versus Performance of PTCA in Patients Without Documented Ischemia) trial is the first randomized study of FFR-guided PCI involving 12 hospitals in Europe and two in Asia.[26] A total of 325 patients were randomly assigned to three groups comprising the Defer group with FFR ≥0.75 (n = 91) in whom PCI was deferred, the Perform group (n = 90) with FFR ≥0.75 in whom PCI was performed and Reference group (n = 144) with FFR <0.75 in whom PCI was performed as originally planned. There was no significant difference in the event-free survival between the Defer and Perform groups during 2- and 5-year follow-up (80% and 73%, p = 0.52), but high incidence of mortality, myocardial infarction or revascularization was noticed in the Perform and Reference groups (p < 0.05). PCI is not recommended for patients with FFR ≥ 0.75 because it has no benefit for patients with hemodynamically insignificant lesions. However, coronary lesions with FFR <0.75 are associated with the greatest risk of developing major adverse cardiac events due to myocardial ischemia caused by functionally significant stenosis.

This study highlights the importance of quantifying the coronary stenosis and corresponding hemodynamic significance.

The multicenter randomized clinical FAME (FFR vs Angiography for Multivessel Evaluation) studies have further confirmed the value of FFR-guided PCI, especially in patients with multivessel CADs.[28,31–34] The FAME trial involved recruiting 1,005 patients with multivessel CAD who were randomly assigned to FFR-guided or angiography-guided PCI. Patients were followed up for 1 year to determine major adverse cardiac events.[32] Results showed FFR-guided PCI group is associated with the saving of healthcare resources and improved outcomes at 1 year when compared with the traditional angiography-guided group. Prevalence of major adverse cardiac events was 13.2% in the FFR-guided group, which is significantly lower than those in the angiography-guided group, which is 18.3% ($p = 0.02$). Mean quality-adjusted life years were higher in the FFR-guided group (0.853 vs 0.838, $p = 0.2$). The mean overall costs at 1 year were significantly lower in the FFR-guided group than those in the angiography-guided group ($14,315 ± 11,109 vs $16,700 ± 11,868; $p < 0.001$). Despite promising outcomes arising from the FAME trial, medical treatment or therapy was not assessed. This has been addressed by the following FAME 2 trials.

The FAME 2 study involved the enrollment of 1,220 patients with stable CAD, with 888 patients randomly assigned to FFR-guided PCI plus medical therapy ($n = 447$) and medical therapy alone groups ($n = 441$).[33,34] The main purpose of this multicenter study is to investigate the superiority of FFR-guided PCI with drug-eluting stents plus best medical therapy over the best available medical therapy alone with regard to the reduction of major adverse cardiac events. With a mean follow-up of 213–214 days for both groups, FFR-guided PCI plus medical therapy group was associated with significantly lower primary end-point event than those in the medical therapy alone group (4.3% vs 12.7%; hazard ratio, 0.3, $p < 0.001$). At the secondary end points, FFR-guided PCI plus medical therapy group also resulted in significantly lower rate of urgent revascularization than those in the medical therapy alone group (1.6% vs 11.1%, hazard ratio, 0.13, $p < 0.001$).[34] At 2 years' follow-up, a significantly lower rate of revascularization was found in the FFR-guided PCI plus medical therapy group as compared to the medical therapy alone

(4.0% vs 16.3%, hazard ratio, 0.23, $p < 0.001$).[33] FFR-guided PCI plus medical therapy improved the clinical outcome when compared to the medical therapy alone.

These FAME studies mainly highlight the limited value of anatomy-based assessment of intermediate coronary lesions for determining functional significance. For example, according to visual estimation, 65% of coronary lesions with 50–70% diameter stenosis were not associated with an abnormal FFR (≤ 0.80), and 20% of lesions with 71–90% diameter stenosis were not associated with an abnormal FFR (Fig. 6.2).[32,35] In patients without hemodynamically stenosis, an excellent 2-year clinical outcome was achieved with the best medical therapy alone, regardless of the degree of coronary stenosis as assessed on coronary angiography. This has been further confirmed by the RIPCORD (Does Routine Pressure Wire Assessment Influence Management Strategy at Coronary Angiography for Diagnosis of Chest Pain) study which assessed the influential role of FFR on patient management.[36] Two hundred patients with stable chest pain were enrolled from 10 cardiology centers in the UK. Management plan comprising medical therapy alone, PCI, coronary artery bypass grafting (CABG) or more information required was assessed in these patients to determine if FFR changed the management strategy when compared to ICA. This study shows that FFR changed the management plan in 26% of the patients whose diagnosis was based on ICA alone. The number of coronary arteries was altered in 64 cases (32%) which were incorrectly diagnosed at ICA. These vessels were found to have significant stenosis upon FFR analysis, thus requiring revascularization. Routine use of FFR has significant clinical value in improving patient management.

6.3 CCTA-Derived FFR: FFR$_{CT}$

Invasive FFR has some limitations that restrict its widespread use in daily clinical practice. It is an invasive procedure as FFR measurement is conducted via pressure guidewire during ICA. It has been reported that only 6% of the PCI procedures in the United States are guided by FFR.[37] This is mainly due to the risk associated with coronary interventional procedures with complications of coronary dissection or occlusion as well as

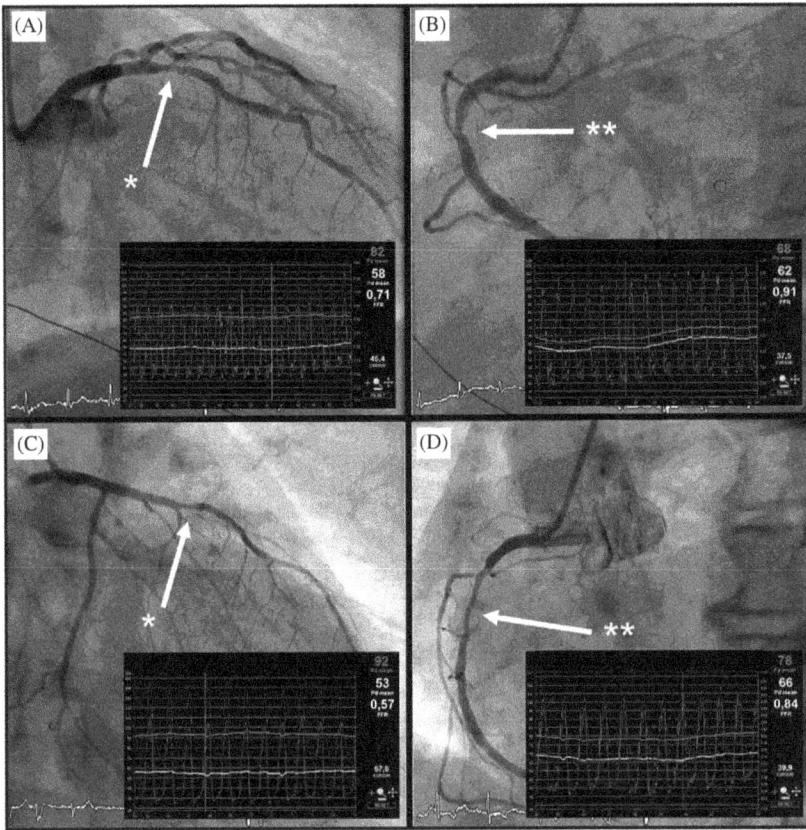

Figure 6.2. Examples of patients with same severity of coronary stenosis on ICA but with different functional importance as assessed by FFR. (A) and (B) ICA shows 50–70% stenosis in the left anterior descending and right coronary arteries as assessed by visual operator's assessment. After the patients were randomized to the FFR-guided arm of the FAME study, the FFR was measured in both arteries. FFR was below the ischemic threshold of 0.80 in the left anterior descending artery (0.71), which was subsequently stented, while FFR of the right coronary artery was 0.91, indicating no functional significance. (C) and (D) Another patient in the FAME study with lumen stenosis between 70 and 90% as assessed by ICA. The left anterior descending lesion was functional significance with FFR of 0.57, and was treated by stent placement, while FFR of the right coronary artery was 0.84. Reprinted with permission from Tonino et al.[35]

cost issue.[38,39] FFR may be estimated/calculated non-invasively from CCTA, leading to the development of FFR_{CT}. There are three steps involved with FFR_{CT} which are discussed in detail below.

The first step in generating FFR_{CT} is to create a highly accurate patient-specific geometric model consisting of the aorta and coronary arteries. This can be achieved with latest multislice CT scanners with improved spatial and temporal resolution, thus enabling acquisition of high-quality CCTA images with minimal artifacts despite high heart rates.[40–42] Once a volumetric model of the coronary artery tree is produced, the second step is to quantify inflow and outflow boundary conditions which represent patient-specific coronary physiology. Normal physiological conditions can be simulated with parameters similar to coronary flow, resistance and pressure under resting conditions and under hyperemic conditions.[43,44] During invasive FFR, hyperemia is done through intravenous injection of adenosine (140 μg/kg of body weight per minute), while for FFR_{CT}, this must be simulated without involving any invasive procedures. The third step is to perform computational fluid dynamics (CFD) simulations through implementation of the Navier–Stokes equations which govern fluid dynamics, allowing for calculation of hemodynamic parameters along the coronary artery model.[45,46] FFR_{CT} is then calculated with the same approach as used in invasive FFR, which is the ratio of mean pressure in the coronary artery distal to the lesion divided by the mean pressure in the aorta during maximal hyperemia in a cardiac cycle. Figure 6.3 shows these steps to calculate FFR_{CT} through coronary CT angiographic data.

6.3.1   Diagnostic Value of FFR_{CT}: Multicenter Results

FFR_{CT} has been shown to improve diagnostic accuracy over CCTA alone for detection of hemodynamic significant coronary stenosis, according to several multicenter studies. Table 6.1 summarizes these multicenter studies with regard to the diagnostic value of FFR_{CT}.

Currently, there are four multicenter reports investigating the diagnostic value of FFR_{CT} in the detection of functional significance of intermediate coronary stenotic lesions when compared to CCTA, namely, DISCOVER-FLOW, NXT, DeFACTO and NOVEL-FLOW.[47–50] The first

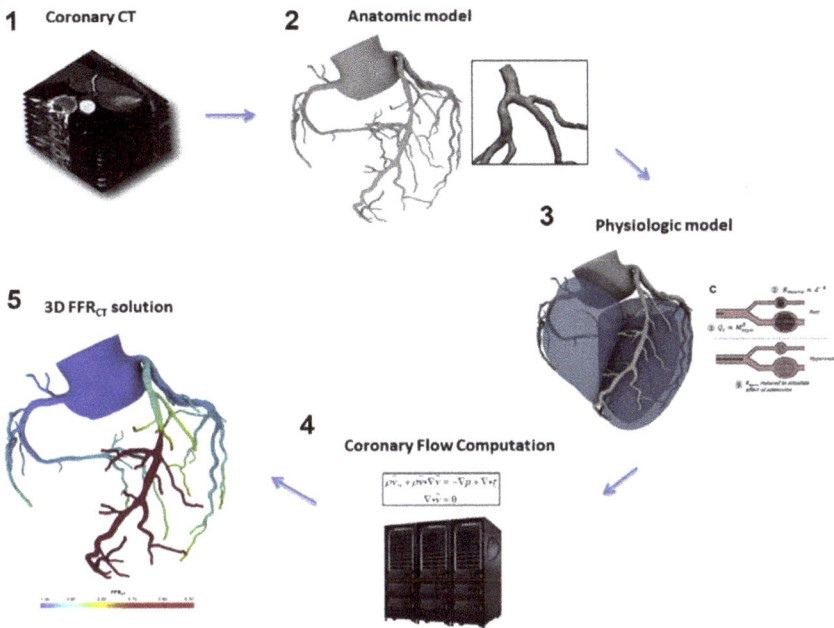

Figure 6.3. Steps to generate FFR$_{CT}$. (1) Coronary CT angiography dataset acquired using standard imaging protocol. (2) Anatomic model of aortic root and coronary arteries including main and side branches. Segmented coronary model allows for construction of tetrahedral mesh, resulting in millions of discrete point for computation of coronary pressure and flow. (3) Physiologic model of coronary tree with specified inflow and outflow boundary conditions. Resting coronary flow is based on myocardial mass, maximal hyperemia is modeled to reflect expected reduction in peripheral resistance resulting from adenosine administration. (4) Computation of coronary pressure and flow by solving the governing equations (Navier–Stokes) of blood flow. (5) 3D solution of FFR through FFR$_{CT}$ throughout the coronary artery tree. Reprinted with permission from Cheruvu *et al.*[43]

three prospective multicenter studies, DISCOVER-FLOW, NXT and DeFACTO are representative studies providing evidence of improved diagnostic performance of FFR$_{CT}$ over conventional CCTA and have been widely reported in the literature. The main findings of these studies include significant improvements in specificity and PPV without change in sensitivity as shown in Table 6.1. CCTA data were transferred to an off-site computational center reporting the FFR$_{CT}$ results (Heart-Flow Inc., Redwood City, California).

Table 6.1. Multicenter studies comparing FFR$_{CT}$ with CCTA with invasive FFR as the gold standard in the diagnosis of CAD.

Diagnostic value CCTA/FFR$_{CT}$	DISCOVER-FLOW[47]		DeFACTO[48]		NXT[49]		NOVEL-FLOW[50]	
	Per-patient assessment	Per-vessel assessment	Per-patient assessment	Per-vessel assessment	Per-patient assessment	Per-vessel assessment	Per-patient assessment	Per-vessel assessment
CCTA ≥ 50%								
Sensitivity	94 (85–99)	91 (81–97)	84 (77–99)	N/A	94 (86–97)	83 (74–89)	84 (76–93)	76 (67–85)
Specificity	25 (13–39)	40 (30–50)	42 (34–51)	N/A	34 (27–41)	60 (56–65)	34 (21–48)	60 (51–68)
PPV	58 (47–68)	47 (37–56)	61 (53–67)	N/A	40 (33–47)	33 (27–39)	66 (56–75)	56 (47–64)
NPV	80 (52–96)	89 (76–96)	72 (61–81)	N/A	92 (83–97)	92 (88–95)	59 (41–78)	79 (71–87)
FFR$_{CT}$ ≤ 0.80								
Sensitivity	93 (82–98)	88 (77–95)	90 (83–95)	80 (73–86)	86 (77–92)	84 (75–89)	93 (87–99)	86 (79–94)
Specificity	82 (68–91)	82 (73–89)	54 (45–63)	61 (54–67)	79 (72–84)	86 (82–89)	75 (62–87)	86 (80–92)
PPV	85 (73–93)	74 (62–84)	67 (60–74)	56 (49–62)	65 (56–74)	61 (53–69)	84 (76–93)	80 (72–88)
NPV	91 (78–98)	92 (85–97)	84 (74–91)	84 (78–89)	93 (87–96)	95 (93–97)	88 (77–98)	90 (85–96)
No. of clinical sites/center, patients and vessels	4 centers from 3 countries 103 patients with 159 vessels		17 centers from 5 countries 252 patients with 408 vessels		10 centers from 8 countries 254 patients with 484 vessels		4 centers from 1 country 117 patients with 218 vessels	

Note: Data are presented as percentages (95% confidence interval), PPV: positive predictive value, NP: negative predictive value, N/A: not available.

DISCOVER-FLOW (Diagnosis of Ischemia-causing Stenoses Obtained Via Non-invasive FFR) was the first multicenter trial that used the first-generation of FFR_{CT} algorithm (version 1.0) for calculating FFR_{CT} results.[47] With sensitivity remaining unchanged, specificity was significantly increased from 40% to 82%, corresponding to CCTA and FFR_{CT}, respectively. The improved diagnostic value of FFR_{CT} also lies in the area under the receiver operating characteristics curve (AUC), which is 0.90 vs 0.75, 0.92 vs 0.70 ($p < 0.05$), on per-patient and per-lesion assessment, respectively. The DeFACTO (Determination of Fractional Flow Reserve by Anatomic CT angiography) was the second multicenter trial following DISCOVER-FLOW, and it involved 17 centers.[48] The second-generation of FFR_{CT} algorithm (version 1.2) was used in this trial, and calculation of FFR_{CT} was performed at the FFR_{CT} core laboratory of Heart-Flow. Although specificity of FFR_{CT} was only 54% as compared to the 42% with CCTA, the AUC of FFR_{CT} was significantly higher than that of CCTA, which is 0.81 vs 0.50, 0.79 vs 0.53 ($p < 0.05$) on per-patient and per-lesion assessment, respectively. The third trial was the NXT (Analysis of Coronary Blood Flow Using CT Angiography: Next Steps) study, in which attention paid to high-quality CCTA images through use of beta-blockers and adjustment of scanning protocols to reduce image noise.[49] The FFR_{CT} algorithm version 1.4 was used in this trial to analyze and calculate FFR_{CT} results. The updated version allows for refinements in CFD simulations such as improvement in coronary lumen boundary and more realistic physiological models. While specificity was increased from 34% to 79%, the AUC was shown to be superior with FFR_{CT}, with AUC of 0.90 vs 0.80, 0.93 vs 0.89 on per-patient and per-lesion assessment ($p < 0.05$), respectively.

The substudy of NXT trial has further confirmed the incremental diagnostic value of FFR_{CT} for the diagnosis of hemodynamically significant coronary stenosis.[51,52] In their recent study, Ko et $al.$ demonstrated that FFR_{CT} offers better diagnostic performance than CCTA and transluminal attenuation gradient (TAG) in 51 patients undergoing 320-slice CCTA with invasive FFR as the reference standard.[51] The sensitivity, specificity, PPV and negative predictive value (NPV) on per-vessel analysis were 79%, 59%, 44% and 87% for CCTA, 58%, 86%, 64% and 83% for TAG, 92%, 79%, 65% and 96% for FFR_{CT}, respectively. The AUC for

FFR_{CT} was 0.93, which is significantly higher than that for CCTA and TAG, which is 0.68 and 0.72 ($p = 0.008 - 0.03$), respectively.

The NOVEL-FLOW study is a recently published multicenter trial which involved four clinical centers in Korea.[50] The purpose of this study was to validate a novel, newly developed CFD technique which is based on vessel-length method for calculation of FFR_{CT}. A total of 117 patients with 218 vessels were included in this retrospective study with CCTA performed on dual-source and 320-slice CT scanners. In this study, 3D patient-specific geometry of coronary arteries were created in combination with the lumped parameter model (LPM), which allows for simulation of micro and venous compartments of the coronary system. In particular, authors developed the vessel-length-based approach to calculate the flow resistances exerted on coronary arteries, which is more efficient than the commonly used time-consuming approach of heart mass and scaling law.[45,53,54]

Figure 6.4 shows the steps to segment coronary artery tree for calculation of FFR_{CT} using this new method employed in the study by Chung *et al.*[50] The first step is to extract the centerlines of the coronary arteries and calculate the summed length of left and right coronary arteries. Then, resistances of coronary arteries are estimated or calculated. The vessel length is inversely proportional to the resistance, meaning the longer the vessel, the lesser the resistance, and thus more blood flow to coronary arteries. The LPM model consists of resistor, capacitor and intramyocardial pressure.[55] The boundary consistency can be ensured by coupling the LPM with 3D CFD coronary model, and thus FFR_{CT} calculation can be obtained in the entire coronary arterial model. To simulate the hyperemic condition (or vasodilation) in the coronary model, coronary microvascular resistance was reduced by up to 25% of the normal one according to the literature.[56] Similar to the previous three multicenter trials, this study shows significant improvements in the diagnostic value of FFR_{CT} over CCTA, with specificity and PPV increased from 34% and 66% to 75% and 84% on per-patient level and 60% and 56% to 86% and 80% on per-vessel, respectively. The AUC of FFR_{CT} was 0.92 and 0.93 on per-patient and per-vessel level, which is significantly higher than that of CCTA, which was 0.68 and 0.74, respectively. Further, the average computational times for CFD simulation were 37.4 min, which is significantly shorter than the previous three multi-center studies, which ranged from 1 to 6 h.

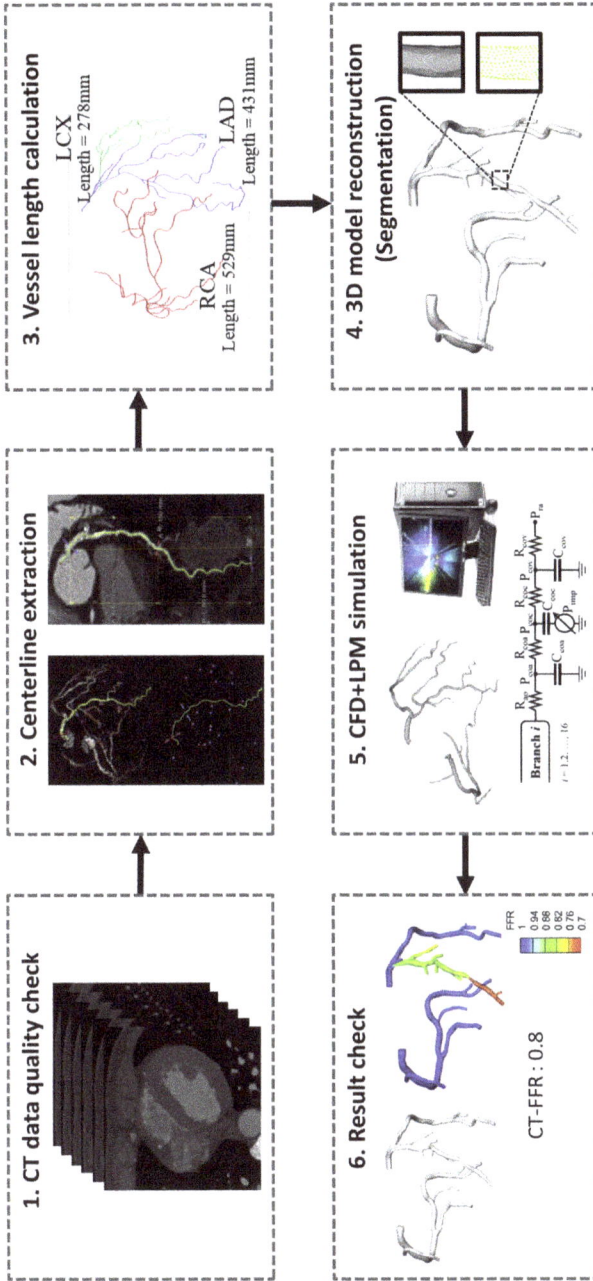

Figure 6.4. Schematic procedure of the simulation for calculation of FFR_{CT} using the vessel-length-based CFD scheme. Reprinted with permission from Chung et al. [50]

6.3.2 Diagnostic Value of FFR$_{CT}$: Single-Center Results

Since FFR$_{CT}$ shows great value in detecting myocardial ischemic coronary lesions, single-center studies are increasingly reported in the literature. Currently, there are around nine studies available on the diagnostic performance of FFR$_{CT}$ in comparison with CCTA.[57–65] Table 6.2 shows study characteristics of these single center studies.

Of these 9 studies, FFR$_{CT}$ was calculated using the Siemens Healthcare cFFR software with version 1.4 used in six studies and a combination of versions 1.4 and 1.7 in one study. The dedicated cFFR software prototype is currently not commercially available. For the remaining two studies, one of them estimated FFR$_{CT}$ with CCTA images transferred to the HeartFlow core laboratory,[59] and another one used dedicated software developed by Toshiba Medical Systems.[60] The main purpose of these single-center studies is to determine the feasibility of performing on-site FFR$_{CT}$ calculation in real clinical practice. Results from these reports are promising, with improved specificity and PPV when compared to CCTA findings which are based on coronary lumen assessment. Good agreement or correlation was found between FFR$_{CT}$ and invasive FFR ($p < 0.001$).

Six of the nine studies compared FFR$_{CT}$ with CCTA when invasive FFR was used as the reference method,[57,60–62,64,65] with diagnostic value assessed on per-vessel level in four studies, and on both per-vessel and per-patient levels in two studies (Table 6.2). It is not surprising to know that the specificity and PPV of CCTA ($\geq$50% stenosis) with reported values ranging from 1.8% to 74% and 37% to 64%, respectively, whereas the corresponding FFR$_{CT}$ results were superior to those of CCTA in these studies, with specificity and PPV ranging from 65% to 91% and 65% to 75%, respectively. Similarly, the AUC was increased from the lowest value of 0.64 with CCTA to the highest 0.92 with FFR$_{CT}$ ($p < 0.05$). In a study by Kruk et al. who reported the lowest specificity and PPV, FFR$_{CT}$ was shown to reclassify 33.3% of all coronary stenoses more accurately than CCTA-based lumen stenosis ($\geq$50%), and up to 11% of stenoses more than other CTA-based criteria (minimum lumen area, quantitative stenosis diameter and stenosis area assessments).[61] This study concludes

Table 6.2. Single-center studies about diagnostic value of FFR$_{CT}$ in the diagnosis of significant coronary stenosis.

Authors and year design	Type of study	CT system	FFR$_{CT}$ software	Cut-off of FFR$_{CT}$/FFR	No. of patients	No. of vessels	CCTA (≥ 50% stenosis) Sen %	Spe %	PPV %	NPV %	FFR$_{CT}$ (≤ 0.80) Sen %	Spe %	PPV %	NPV %	AUC CCTA	FFR$_{CT}$
Coenen et al.[57]	Retrospective and observational	64/128-slice	cFFR v 1.4	≤ 0.80	106	189	81 (71–89)	38 (29–47)	49 (40–58)	73 (60–84)	88 (78–94)	65 (55–74)	65 (55–74)	88 (79–94)	0.64	0.83
De Geer et al.[58]*	Retrospective	128-slice	cFFR v 1.4/ v 1.7	≤ 0.80	21	23	N/A	N/A	N/A	N/A	83/83	76/80	56/63	93/93	N/A	N/A
Kawaji et al.[59]	Prospective, cross-sectional	320-slice	HeartFlow lab	≤ 0.80	43	70	N/A	N/A	N/A	N/A	93	52	57	92	N/A	0.87
Ko et al.[60]	Prospective, cross-sectional	320-slice	Toshiba CT-FFR	≤ 0.80	42	78	79 (54–93)	74 (58–86)	60 (39–78)	88 (71–96)	78 (52–93)	87 (71–95)	74 (49–90)	89 (74–96)	0.77	0.88
Kruk et al.[61]*	Prospective, cross-sectional	128-slice	cFFR v 1.4	≤ 0.80	90	96	100/100	1.8/2.0	43/46	100/100	76/76	72/71	67/69	80/78	0.66	0.84
Renker et al.[62]*	Retrospective	64/128-slice	cFFR v 1.4	≤ 0.80	53	67	90 (68–98/94 (70–99)	34 (21–49)/32 (18–50)	37 (23–52)/38 (23–54)	89 (65–98)/92 (64–99)	85 (62–97)/94 (70–99)	85 (72–94)/84 (68–94)	71 (49–87)/71 (48–89)	93 (81–98)/97 (84–99)	0.72/0.78	0.92/0.91
Tesche et al.[63]	Retrospective	64/128-slice	cFFR v 1.4	≤ 0.80	37	37	N/A	N/A	N/A	N/A	100 (55–100)	90 (69–97)	74 (33–95)	100 (82–100)	N/A	0.85
Wang et al.[64]	Retrospective	64/128-slice	cFFR v 1.4	≤ 0.80	32	32	100 (59–100)	54 (33–73)	42 (21–66)	100 (71–100)	100 (54–100)	91 (71–98)	75 (35–96)	100 (83–100)	N/A	0.91
Yang et al.[65]	Prospective, cross-sectional	128-slice	cFFR v 1.4	≤ 0.80	72	138	94 (84–98)	66 (55–76)	64 (52–75)	94 (8–98)	87 (75–94)	77 (66–85)	71 (58–81)	90 (80–96)	0.86	0.89

Notes: *Indicates studies with reported CCTA and /or FFR$_{CT}$ results which were based on per-lesion/or per-vessel and per-patient assessment. For the remaining studies, diagnostic value was based on per-vessel assessment. CCTA — coronary CT angiography, N/A — not available, PPV — positive predictive value, NPV — negative predictive value; Sen-sensitivity, Spe-specificity.

that FFR_{CT} may confidently discriminate ischemic from non-ischemic stenoses in about 50% of patients with intermediate coronary stenosis, thus having significant clinical value of saving these patients from further functional testing, although results need to be validated by large cohort of studies.

Wang *et al.* in their study conducted analysis of diagnostic value of various quantitative stenosis predictors consisting of coronary diameter stenosis, lesion length/minimal lumen diameter (MLD[4]), TAG and corrected coronary opacification (CCO) with results compared to FFR_{CT} for detection of significant coronary stenosis.[64] Sensitivity, specificity, PPV and NPV of FFR_{CT} were 100%, 91%, 75% and 100%, which is significantly higher than those of CCTA (≥50% stenosis) and TAG (≤ −1.51 HU/mm), with corresponding values being 100%, 54%, 42% and 100%, 37%, 58%, 23% and 73%, but similar to those of CCO (>0.184) and LL/MLD[4] (>3.86), which were 66%, 88%, 57% and 92%, 85%, 92%, 75% and 95%, respectively. The AUC of FFR_{CT} was 0.91, which is significantly higher than that of TAG, which was 0.67 ($p = 0.013$), but was not significantly different from that of CCO and LL/MLD,[4] which had values of 0.85 and 0.88 ($p = 0.419 - 0.819$).

The other three studies only reported diagnostic performance of FFR_{CT} in detecting hemodynamically significant coronary lesions compared with invasive FFR without analyzing diagnostic value of CCTA.[58,59,63] De Geer *et al.* only analyzed 21 patients with inclusion of 23 vessels with the aim of showing on-site efficient calculation of FFR_{CT} with results compared to invasive FFR.[58] The mean time for FFR_{CT} and complete FFR_{CT} post-processing was 3 min 28 s and 45 min, respectively, which is consistent with other single-center reports, but apparently much shorter than that with off-site estimation at the HeartFlow core laboratory (1–4 h for complete FFR_{CT} post-processing, and around 24 h including data transfer from the clinical centers to the HeartFlow laboratory). This pilot study shows the rapid post-processing of CCTA data with subsequent computation of FFR_{CT} through use of the workstation-based software.

Although Kawaji *et al.* only focused on the diagnostic value of FFR_{CT} in the real clinical world, they did assess the effect of calcified plaques on FFR_{CT} in their study comprising 43 patients with analysis of 70 vessels.[59]

Good correlation was found between FFR_{CT} and invasive FFR even in patients with calcium score >1,000 ($p < 0.001$). On per-vessel level, sensitivity, specificity, PPV and NPV of FFR_{CT} were 100%, 62%, 62% and 100% in patients with severely calcified plaques, and 91%, 50%, 55% and 90% in patients without severely calcified plaques. This study confirms the diagnostic performance of FFR_{CT} for detection of hemodynamically significant CAD, regardless of severity of the calcification in coronary arteries.

In their recent study, Tesche *et al.* further validated the diagnostic ability of FFR_{CT} and other quantitative stenosis predictors for detecting lesion-specific ischemia.[63] In addition to CCO and TAG, authors included remodeling index, total plaque volume (TPV), calcified and non-calcified plaque volume (CPV and NCPV), and vessel volume (VV) with results compared to FFR_{CT}. At the per-vessel level, FFR_{CT} has the highest specificity and PPV, which were 90% and 74% (Fig. 6.5). This is significantly higher than those of TAG, remodeling index, VV and CPV, which were 56% and 22%, 54% and 53%, 66% and 22%, 53% and 21%, but is similar to those of CCO, TPV and NCPV, with corresponding values being 86% and 55%, 74% and 43%, 81% and 48%, respectively. The AUC of FFR_{CT} was 0.85, similar to that of CCO, TPV and NCPV, which was 0.82, 0.78 and 0.80, respectively, but significantly higher than that of TAG, remodeling index, VV and CPV, which was 0.64, 0.58, 0.73 and 0.73, respectively (Fig. 6.6). The authors concluded that FFR_{CT} along with other parameters including CCO, TPV and NCPV allow for determination of significant coronary stenoses. This is consistent with findings from Wang *et al.*'s study,[64] with both of them highlighting the limited diagnostic value of CCTA-based coronary lumen assessment, while FFR_{CT} demonstrated the most significant discriminatory ability in diagnosing ischemic coronary stenoses.

6.3.3 Diagnostic Value of FFR_{CT}: Systematic Review and Meta-analysis

Due to increasing reports on the clinical application of FFR_{CT} in identifying significant coronary stenosis, several systematic reviews and meta-analyses are available in the literature in recent years. So far, there are seven systematic reviews/meta-analyses reporting the diagnostic perfor-

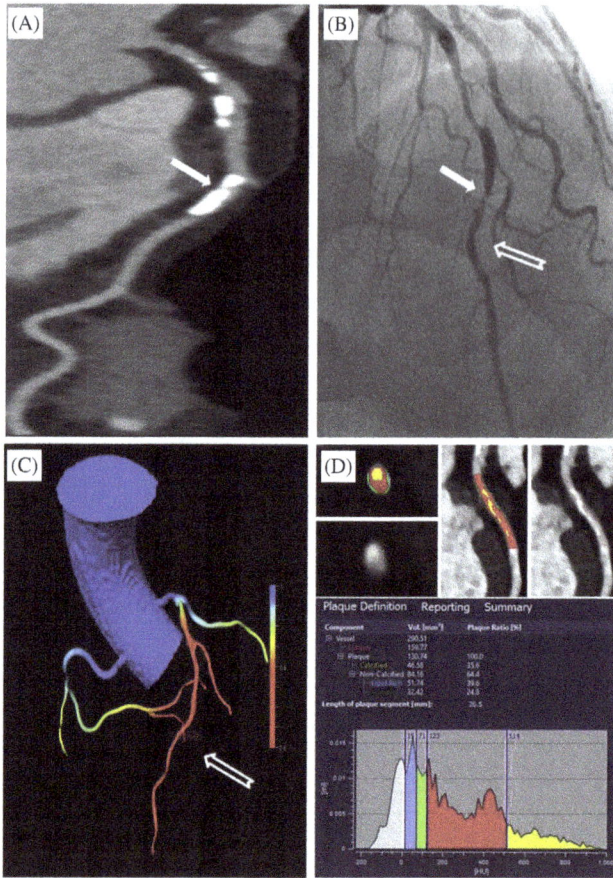

Figure 6.5. (A) Coronary CT angiography shows significant stenosis of the left anterior descending coronary artery due to mixed calcified plaque (arrow). (B) ICA confirms significant stenosis. (C) FFR$_{CT}$ with color-coded 3D mesh shows FFR value of 0.73, indicating ischemic lesion. (D) Color-coded plaque assessment of the corresponding stenosis. Reprinted with permission from Tesche *et al.*[63]

mance of FFR$_{CT}$ in comparison with CCTA or other imaging modalities with invasive FFR as the reference standard.[66–72] Table 6.3 summarizes the summed diagnostic value according to these studies. As shown in the table, six of them reported the diagnostic value of FFR$_{CT}$ vs CCTA in the diagnosis of hemodynamic significance of CAD, while in the remaining

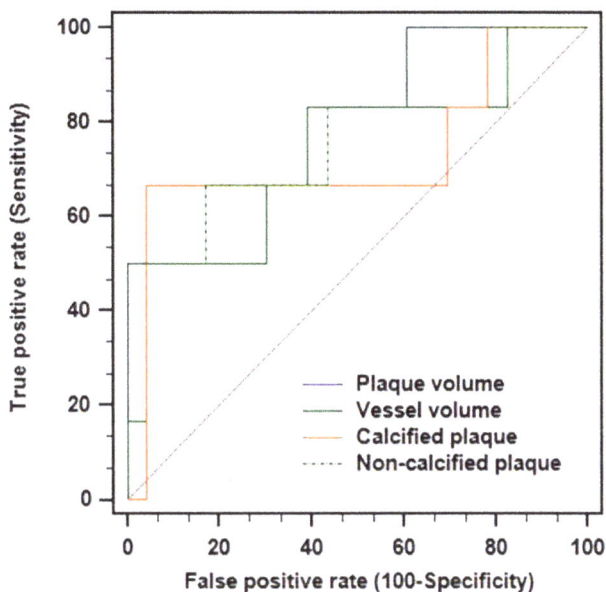

Parameter	AUC	95%CI	p-value
TPV	0.783	0.59-0.91	0.013
VV	0.732	0.54-0.88	0.09
CPV	0.725	0.53-0.87	0.14
NCPV	0.797	0.61-0.92	0.009

Figure 6.6. Area under the curve of receiver operating characteristics showed diagnostic value of morphological predictors for hemodynamic significance. CPV-calcified plaque volume, NCPV-non-calcified plaque volume, TPV-total plaque volume, VV-vessel volume. Reprinted with permission from Tesche *et al.*[63]

study,[71] only diagnostic value of FFR$_{CT}$ was available. The three multi-center studies including DISCOVER-FLOW, NXT and DeFACTO were included in two of the meta-analyses,[70,72] whereas multicenter and single center studies were analyzed in the other five studies with number of studies ranging from 5 to 16 for CCTA, 3 to 8 for FFR$_{CT}$.

Results of these analyses provide further evidence about the improved diagnostic performance of FFR$_{CT}$ over CCTA. On per-vessel level analysis, the pooled specificity and PPV ranged from 50% to 65%, 38% to 48% for CCTA, and this increased to more than 70% (between 71% and 79%),

Table 6.3.   Summary of diagnostic value of FFR_{CT} in the diagnosis of significant coronary stenosis based on systematic reviews and meta-analyses.

Authors	No. of studies	No. of patients/ vessels	Diagnostic value of CCTA on per-vessel/per-patient level (%)				Diagnostic value of FFR_{CT} on per-vessel/per-patient level (%)				AUC	
			Sensitivity	Specificity	PPV	NPV	Sensitivity	Specificity	PPV	NPV	CCTA	FFR_{CT}
Baumann et al.[66]	5	765/1306	85 (78–91)/ 90 (81–100)	50 (31–68)/ 35 (24–47)	39 (28–50)/ 51 (31–71)	87 (72–100)/ 83 (65–100)	84 (78–89)/ 89 (84–95)	75 (52–97)/ 70 (45–96)	65 (52–78)/ 69 (56–83)	90 (81–99)/ 90 (81–99)	0.74/0.74 (0.63–0.86)/ 0.62–0.85	0.9/0.87 (0.82–0.98)/ (0.77–0.96)
Danad et al.[67]	10/3	609/694 1050/2085	91 (88–93)/ 90 (86–93)	58 (55–61)/ 39 (34–44)	N/A	N/A	83 (78–87)/ 90 (85–93)	78 (78–81)/ 71 (63–85)	N/A	N/A	0.85/0.57	0.92/0.94
Ding et al.[68]	16/8	901/1319 1380/2156	87 (85–89)/ 91 (88–93)	63 (60–65)/ 61 (58–65)	N/A	N/A	82 (79–86)/ 90 (86–93)	79 (76–82)/ 73 (68–77)	N/A	N/A	0.85/0.91	0.90/0.96
Gonzalez et al.[69]	9/4	1039/662 1239/714	89 (86–91)/ 92 (88–98)	65 (62–67)/ 43 (38–47)	48 (38–58)/ 57 (51–64)	94 (82–94)/ 87 (78–94)	83 (79–87)/ 90 (85–93)	77 (74–80)/ 72 (67–76)	63 (52–72)/ 70 (58–82)	91 (79–100)/ 90 (84–95)	N/A	N/A
Li et al.[70]	3	753/1050	83 (78–86)/ 89 (85–93)	56 (51–60)/ 35 (30–41)	38 (33–44)/ 52 (47–56)	92 (89–95)/ 81 (73–87)	83 (78–86)/ 89 (85–93)	78 (75–81)/ 71 (65–75)	61 (56–65)/ 70 (65–75)	92 (89–94)/ 90 (85–93)	0.74	0.88/0.89
Wu et al.[71]	7	833/1377	N/A	N/A	N/A	N/A	84 (80–87)/ 89 (85–93)	76 (67–83)/ 76 (64–84)	N/A	N/A	N/A	0.86/0.90 (0.83–0.89)/ (0.87–0.92)
Xu et al.[72]	3	609/1050	81 (80–91)/ 89 (85–93)	56 (51–60)/ 35 (30–41)	39 (34–44)/ 51 (46–56)	93 (89–95)/ 81 (74–87)	83 (78–87)/ 89 (85–93)	78 (75–81)/ 71 (65–75)	61 (56–66)/ 70 (65–75)	92 (89–94)/ 90 (86–93)	N/A	N/A

Notes: AUC: area under the curve of receiving operative characteristics; CCTA: coronary CT angiography; N/A: not available; PPV: positive predictive value; NPV: negative predictive value. Danad et al., Ding et al., Gonzalez et al., 10, 16 and 9 studies for CCTA, and 3, 8 and 4 for FFR_{CT}.

61% to 65% for FFR_{CT}, respectively. On per-patient level analysis, the pooled specificity and PPV ranged from 35% to 61%, 51% to 57% for CCTA, and this increased to more than 70% (between 71% and 76%), 69% to 70% for FFR_{CT}, respectively. In the study showing only diagnostic value of FFR_{CT},[71] the summed specificity was 76% on per-vessel and per-patient assessments. The AUC of ROC analysis was available only in four studies, with the mean value of FFR_{CT} significantly higher than that of CCTA ($p < 0.05$).

In addition to CCTA vs FFR_{CT}, other functional imaging modalities were included in the analysis in two studies. Gonzalez *et al.* in their study compared CCTA, CT perfusion (CTP) and FFR_{CT} for assessment of functional myocardial ischemia, with invasive FFR as the reference standard.[69] On per-vessel analysis, pooled specificity and PPV were 76% (72–80%) and 61% (46–75%), and 77% (74–80%) and 63% (52–72%) for CTP and FFR_{CT}, respectively, which is significantly higher than those of CCTA, which were 65% (62–67%) and 48% (38–58%). Similar findings were noted on per-patient analysis, with pooled specificity and PPV being 77% (66–85%) and 83% (75–92%), and 72% (67–76%) and 70% (58–82%) for CTP and FFR_{CT}, respectively, and this is significantly higher than those of CCTA, which were 43% (38–47%) and 57% (51–64%). They concluded that both CTP and FFR_{CT} improved specificity and PPV of CCTA on per-vessel and per-patient analysis for detecting ischemic coronary stenoses, although CTP was associated with higher radiation dose when compared to CCTA (9.6 vs 3.5 mSv).

In their recent report, Danad and colleagues conducted a meta-analysis of diagnostic performance of various imaging modalities including single-photon emission computed tomography (SPECT), stress echocardiography (SE), CCTA, ICA, FFR_{CT} and cardiac magnetic resonance imaging (MRI) when compared with invasive FFR.[67] So far, this analysis represents the most comprehensive analysis of studies involving different imaging modalities in the detection of functional significance of coronary stenoses. A total of 23 studies were eligible in the analysis, comprising 10 CCTA studies (1,167 patients), 3 SE (141 patients), 3 FFR_{CT} (609 patients), 6 ICA (2,610 patients), 6 SPECT (282 patients) and 4 MRI studies (132 patients). On per-vessel analysis, pooled sensitivity and specificity were 91% (88–93%) and 58% (55–61%) for CCTA, 83%

(78–87%) and 78% (78–81%) for FFR_{CT}, 71% (69–74%) and 66% (64–68%) for ICA, 91% (84–95%) and 85% (79–89%) for MRI, and 57% (49–64%) and 75% (69–80%) for SPECT, respectively. On per-patient analysis, pooled sensitivity and specificity were 90% (86–93%) and 39% (34–44%) for CCTA, 77% (61–88%) and 75% (63–85%) for SE, 90% (85–93%) and 71% (65–75%) for FFR_{CT}, 69% (65–75%) and 67% (63–71%) for ICA, 90% (75–97%) and 94% (79–99%) for MRI, and 70% (59–80%) and 78% (68–87%) for SPECT, respectively. Their analysis shows that MRI has the highest diagnostic performance of detecting ischemia-causing CAD, while diagnostic performance of ICA, SE and SPECT was quite low. Both CCTA and FFR_{CT} have high sensitivity, but FFR_{CT} demonstrates improved specificity over CCTA on both per-vessel and per-patient analysis. The findings of this analysis need to be interpreted with caution due to limited number of studies in the analysis, especially the very small number of studies for SE, MRI and FFR_{CT}.

Apart from these systematic reviews and meta-analyses, several general review articles also provide an excellent overview of the clinical applications of FFR_{CT} in providing physiological assessment of significant coronary stenosis. Readers can refer to these review articles for more details.[14,22,43,46,73–77]

6.3.4 Diagnostic Value of FFR_{CT}: Limitations and Challenges

Despite promising results available in the current literature, either from studies based on multicenter trials or single-center reports, as well as some meta-analyses, there are some limitations with use of FFR_{CT} which should be acknowledged. First, with CCTA data transferred to an off-site workstation at the HeartFlow, the turnaround time is about 24 h, which is impractical for routine clinical application of FFR_{CT}. The mean duration of estimating FFR_{CT} is around 30 min with the use of Siemens cFFR or Toshiba CT-FFR when compared to the 1–4 h with use of HeartFlow FFR_{CT}.[60] However, these software tools, in particular the commonly used Siemens cFFR is a prototype version and not commercially available, which limits the studies to only a few clinical centers. Future versions including technical developments are expected to improve the diagnostic ability.

Second, there is a lack of evidence to prove how FFR_{CT} changes patient's managements and clinical outcomes as majority of current studies are cross-sectional single-center studies (either prospective or retrospective in terms of study design); therefore, there is a strong demand for cohort studies with follow-up data. Adding FFR_{CT} to CCTA is expected to significantly improve the specificity and PPV because of the coupling of anatomic and functional approaches. This is confirmed by a recently published PLATFORM (Prospective LongitudinAl Trial of FFR_{CT}: Outcome and Resource Impacts).[78] In this multicenter prospective trial, Douglas *et al.* recruited 584 patients with new onset chest pain from 11 clinical sites. Of the patients in this cohort, 287 received usual testing and 297 received CCTA/FFR_{CT} as a diagnostic testing. Patients were followed up at 90 days to determine the prevalence of cardiac events rates (death, myocardial infarction and unplanned revascularization) in these two groups. Results demonstrated the superiority of CCTA/FFR_{CT} in patient care and management with a cancellation of 61% ICA procedures in patients after receiving CCTA/FFR_{CT}.[78,79] This study further confirms the limited value of CCTA alone as represented by the PROMISE trial, which showed the increased rate of invasive ICA by 50% when CCTA was used as a test to determine significant coronary stenosis in comparison with functional testing.[9] Further studies with long-term follow-up are needed to determine the additional value of FFR_{CT} in guiding patient management.

Third, image quality of original source CCTA data directly affects the calculation of FFR_{CT} values. It has been reported that imaging artifacts, especially due to misalignment, negatively influence the diagnostic performance of FFR_{CT}. More than 10% of patients were found to be unevaluable due to artifacts or severe coronary calcification, according to some single-center and multicenter studies.[48,49,65] Thus, using a high-end CT scanner is preferable to enable acquisition of high-resolution CCTA images.

Finally, radiation dose associated with CCTA including FFR_{CT} should not be ignored due to the increasing use of CCTA-derived FFR_{CT}. Although FFR_{CT} does not directly affect patient's data since it is calculated from CCTA data, the image processing and calculation process requires satisfactory CCTA data which is essential for the generation of high-quality coronary model for computational simulations. Bilbey *et al.*

in their clinical model used a sample of 1,000 stable, symptomatic patients with stable CAD and modeled four treatment pathways based on the first non-invasive diagnostic imaging performed: dobutamine echocardiography, SPECT, CCTA and CCTA /FFR$_{CT}$.[80] The cardiac events rate (death/ myocardial infarction) at 1-year estimation with different pretest probability of CAD was determined based on different imaging pathways. Their analysis showed that stress echo resulted in the lowest radiation dose levels of 5.4 mSv (including 4.0 mSv from ICA and 1.4 mSv from PCI), while SPECT imaging test had the highest radiation exposure of 26.5 mSv, while CCTA and FFR$_{CT}$ were associated with 14.2 and 9.7 mSv for the average cumulative dose. For a disease prevalence of 10% and 90%, FFR$_{CT}$ was associated with radiation dose ranging from 6.4 to 16.2 mSv, which is higher than that of stress echo (4.2–7.7 mSv), but significantly lower than that of CCTA (11.9–18.7 mSv) and SPECT (25.4–28.7 mSv). The combination of CCTA+ FFR$_{CT}$ led to the lowest 1-year event rate (1.44% for 10% disease prevalence, and 4.40% for 90% disease prevalence), while the highest event rate was seen in stress echo (2.84% and 5.23% for 10% and 90% disease prevalence, respectively). Further, CCTA+ FFR$_{CT}$ pathway resulted in lower cost with an average of $4,384 per patient, slightly higher than that of stress echo ($3,706), but significantly lower than that of CCTA and SPECT ($6,835 and $6,757) respectively. This analysis suggests that incorporation of FFR$_{CT}$ into CCTA diagnostic pathway reduced radiation dose with improved clinical outcomes, although randomized controlled trials are needed to confirm these findings.[81]

6.4 Summary and Conclusion

CCTA-derived FFR$_{CT}$ has represented a paradigm shift in diagnosing hemodynamically significant coronary stenosis by showing accuracy and improved diagnostic value in detecting lesion-specific ischemia. FFR$_{CT}$ has overcome the limitations of CCTA due to its low diagnostic accuracy in detecting functional significance of coronary stenosis. Evidence from the current literature based on multicenter and single-center studies supports the use of FFR$_{CT}$ in clinical practice when assessing coronary artery lesions. However, more research is needed before it is recommended in daily practice due to several reasons. First, although FFR_{CT} significantly improves specificity and PPV when compared to CCTA, its diagnostic value is moderate with reported specificity and PPV less than 80%. Therefore, further evidence is required to demonstrate its high diagnostic performance. Second, developments in software tools for calculation of FFR_{CT} represent another challenge, as currently available software algorithms belong to the prototype which is not commercially available. HeartFlow has received FDA approval; however, data transfer to an off-site workstation for FFR_{CT} estimation is not a realistic approach for daily clinical practice. Thus, only a small number of studies are available in the literature, despite the introduction of FFR_{CT} in clinical practice more than 6 years ago. Third, acquisition of high-quality CCTA datasets with minimal artifacts is essential to guarantee the final FFR_{CT} results. This is possible with latest multislice CT scanners with superior spatial and temporal resolution. Finally, active collaboration between clinicians, medical imaging scientists, computer scientists and biomedical engineers plays an important role in assuring successful implementation of this novel technique in the diagnostic assessment of CAD. With more research being conducted on a large scale, FFR_{CT} will continue to improve our understanding of pathophysiology of CAD and serve as a reliable tool to provide more accurate analysis of coronary lesions through which effective treatment strategies can be established.

References

1. Miller JM, Rochitte CE, Dewey M *et al.* (2008) Diagnostic performance of coronary angiography by 64-row CT. *N Engl J Med* **359**: 2324–2336.
2. Meijboom WB, Meijs MF, Schuijf JD *et al.* (2008) Diagnostic accuracy of 64-slice computed tomography coronary angiography: a prospective, multicenter, multivendor study. *J Am Coll Cardiol* **52**: 2135–2144.
3. Sun Z, Choo GH, Ng KH. (2012) Coronary CT angiography: current status and continuing challenges. *Br J Radiol* **85**: 495–510.
4. Sun Z, Lin C. (2014) Diagnostic value of 320-slice coronary CT angiography in coronary artery disease: a systematic review and meta-analysis. *Curr Med Imaging Rev* **10**: 272–280.
5. Sun Z, Wan YL, Hsieh IC, Liu YC, Wen MS. (2013) Coronary CT angiography in the diagnosis of coronary artery disease. *Curr Med Imaging Rev* **9**: 184–193.

6. Sun Z, Cao Y, Li H. (2011) Multislice CT angiography in the diagnosis of coronary artery disease. *J Geriatr Cardiol* **8**: 104–113.
7. Gaudio C, Pelliccia F, Evangelista A, Tanzilli G, Paravati V *et al.* (2013) 320-row computed tomography coronary angiography vs. conventional coronary angiography in patients with suspected coronary artery disease: a systematic review and meta-analysis. *Int J Cardiol* **168**: 1562–1564.
8. Li S, Ni Q, Wu H, Peng L, Dong R *et al.* (2013) Diagnostic accuracy of 320-slice computed tomography angiography for detection of coronary artery stenosis: meta-analysis. *Int J Cardiol* **168**: 2699–2705.
9. Douglas PS, Hoffmann U, Patel MR *et al.* (2015) Outcomes of anatomical versus functional testing for coronary artery disease. *N Engl J Med* **372**: 1291–1300.
10. Meijboom WB, Van Mieghem CA, van Pelt N *et al.* (2008) Comprehensive assessment of coronary artery stenoses: computed tomography coronary angiography versus conventional coronary angiography and correlation with fractional flow reserve in patients with stable angina. *J Am Coll Cardiol* **52**: 636–643.
11. Schuijf JD, Wijns W, Jukema JW *et al.* (2006) Relationship between noninvasive coronary angiography with multi-slice computed tomography and myocardial perfusion imaging. *J Am Coll Cardiol* **48**: 2508–2514.
12. Cheng V, Gutstein A, Wolak A, *et al.* (2008) Moving beyond binary grading of coronary arterial stenoses on coronary computed tomographic angiography: insights for the imager and referring clinician. *JACC: Cardiovasc Imaging* **1**(4): 460–471.
13. Min JK, Berman D. (2009) Anatomic and functional assessment of coronary artery disease: convergence of 2 aims in a single setting. *Circ Cardiovasc Imaging* **2**(3): 163–165.
14. Pang CL, Alcock R, Pilkington N, Reis T, Roobottom C. (2016) Determining the haemodynamic significance of arterial stenosis: the relationship between CT angiography, computational fluid dynamics, and non-invasive fractional flow reserve. *Clin Radiol* **71**: 750–757.
15. Zhang LJ, Wu SY, Wang J *et al.* (2010) Diagnostic accuracy of dual-source CT coronary angiography: the effect of average heart rate, heart rate variability, and calcium score in a clinical perspective. *Acta Radiol* **51**: 727–740.
16. Gang S, Min L, Li L, Guo-Ying L, Lin X, Qun J, Hua Z. (2012) Evaluation of CT coronary artery angiography with 320-row detector CT in a high-risk population. *Br J Radiol* **85**: 562–570.
17. Uehara M, Funabashi N, Takaoka H, Fujimoto Y, Kobayashi Y. (2014) False-positive findings in 320-slice cardiac CT for detection of severe coronary stenosis in comparison with invasive coronary angiography indicate poor prognosis for occurrence of MACE. *Int J Cardiol* **172**: 235–237.
18. Sun Z, Abdul Aziz Y, Ng KH. (2012) Coronary CT angiography: how should physicians use it widely and when do physicians request it appropriately? *Eur J Radiol* **81**: e684–e687.

19. Meijboom WB, Van Mieghem CA, Mollet NR *et al.* (2007) 64-slice computed tomography coronary angiography in patients with high, intermediate, or low pretest probability of significant coronary artery disease. *J Am Coll Cardiol* **50**: 1469–1475.

20. Patel MR, Peterson ED, Dai D *et al.* (2010) Low diagnostic yield of elective coronary angiography. *N Engl J Med* **362**: 886–895.

21. Toth G, Hamilos M, Pyxaras S *et al.* (2014) Evolving concepts of angiogram: fractional flow reserve discordances in 4000 coronary stenoses. *Eur Heart J* **35**: 2831–2838.

22. Corcoran D, Hennigan B, Berry C. (2017) Fractional flow reserve: a clinical perspective. *Int J Cardiovasc Imaging* **33**: 961–974.

23. Task Force Members, Montalescot G, Sechtem U, Achenbach S, Andreotti F, Arden C *et al.* (2013) ESC guidelines on the management of stable coronary artery disease: the Task Force on the management of stable coronary artery disease of the European Society of Cardiology. *Eur Heart J* **34**: 2949–3003.

24. Pijls NH, De Bruyne B, Peels K *et al.* (1996) Measurement of fractional flow reserve to assess the functional severity of coronary-artery stenoses. *N Engl J Med* **334**: 1703–1708.

25. Bech GJ, De Bruyne B, Pijls NH *et al.* (2001) Fractional flow reserve to determine the appropriateness of angioplasty in moderate coronary stenosis: a randomized trial. *Circulation* **103**: 2928–2934.

26. Pijls NH, van Schaardenburgh P, Manoharan G *et al.* (2007) Percutaneous coronary intervention of functionally nonsignificant stenosis: 5-year follow-up of the DEFER Study. *J Am Coll Cardiol* **49**: 2105–2111.

27. Zimmermann FM, Ferrara A, Johnson NP *et al.* (2015) Deferral vs. performance of percutaneous coronary intervention of functionally non-significant coronary stenosis: 15-year follow-up of the DEFER trial. *Eur Heart J* **36**: 3182–3188.

28. Tonino PA, De Bruyne B, Pijls NH *et al.* (2009) Fractional flow reserve versus angiography for guiding percutaneous coronary intervention. *N Engl J Med* **360**: 213–224.

29. Pijls NH, Fearon WF, Tonino PA *et al.* (2010) Fractional flow reserve versus angiography for guiding percutaneous coronary intervention in patients with multivessel coronary artery disease: 2-year follow-up of the FAME (Fractional Flow Reserve Versus Angiography for Multivessel Evaluation) study. *J Am Coll Cardiol* **56**: 177–184.

30. van Nunen LX, Zimmermann FM, Tonino PA *et al.* (2015) Fractional flow reserve versus angiography for guidance of PCI in patients with multivessel coronary artery disease (FAME): 5-year follow-up of a randomised controlled trial. *Lancet* **386**: 1853–1860.

31. Fearon WF, Tonino PA, De Bruyne B, Siebert U, Pijls NH, FAME Study Investigators. (2007) Rationale and design of the Fractional Flow Reserve Versus Angiography for Multivessel Evaluation (FAME) study. *Am Heart J* **154**: 632–636.

32. Fearon WF, Bornschein B, Tonino PA *et al.* (2010) Fractional flow reserve versus angiography for multivessel evaluation (FAME) study investigators. Economic evaluation of fractional flow reserve-guided percutaneous coronary intervention in patients with multivessel disease. *Circulation* **122**: 2545–2550.

33. De Bruyne B, Pijls NH, Kalesan B *et al.* (2012) FAME 2 Trial Investigators. Fractional flow reserve-guided PCI versus medical therapy in stable coronary disease. *N Engl J Med* **367**: 991–1001.

34. De Bruyne B, Fearon WF, Oijls NHJ *et al.* (2014) Fractional flow reserve-guided PCI for stable coronary artery disease. *N Engl J Med* **371**: 1208–1217.

35. Tonino PAL, Fearon WF, De Bruyne B *et al.* (2010) Angiography versus functional severity of coronary artery stenoses in the FAME study. *J Am Coll Cardiol* **55**: 2816–2821.

36. Curzen N, Rana O, Nicholas Z *et al.* (2014) Does routine pressure wire assessment influence management strategy at coronary angiography for diagnosis of chest pain? The RIPORD study. *Circ Cardiovasc Interv* **7**: 248–255.

37. Kleiman NS. (2011) Bringing it all together: integration of physiology with anatomy during cardiac catheterization. *J Am Coll Cardiol* **58**: 1219–1221.

38. Morris PD, van de Vosse FN, Lawford PV, Hose DR, Gunn JP. (2015) "Virtual" (computed) fractional flow reserve: current challenges and limitations. *JACC Cardiovasc Interv* **8**: 1009–1017.

39. Precious B, Blanke P, Norgaard BL, Min JK, Leipsic J. (2015) Fractional flow reserve modeled from resting coronary CT angiography: state of the science. *AJR Am J Roentgenol* **204**: W243–W248.

40. Mangold S, Wichmann JL, Schoepf UJ *et al.* (2017) Diagnostic accuracy of coronary CT angiography using 3rd-generation dual-source CT and automated tube voltage selection: clinical application of a non-obese and obese patient population. *Eur Radiol* **27**: 2298–2308.

41. Liang J, Wang H, Xu L *et al.* (2017) Impact of SSF on diagnostic performance of coronary computed tomography angiography within 1 heart beat in patients with high heart rate using a 256-row detector computed tomography. *J Comput Assist Tomogr* Jul 13. doi: 10.1097/RCT.0000000000000641.

42. Liang J, Wang H, Xu L *et al.* (2017) Diagnostic performance of 256-row coronary CT angiography in patients with high heart rates within a single cardiac cycle: a preliminary study. *Clin Radiol* **72**: 694.e7–694.e14.

43. Cheruvu C, Naoum C, Blanke P *et al.* (2016) Beyond stenosis with fractional flow reserve via computed tomography and advanced plaque analyses for the diagnosis of lesion-specific ischemia. *Can J Cardiol* **32**: 1315.e1–1315.e9.

44. Pijls NH, De Bruyne B. (1998) Coronary pressure measurement and fractional flow reserve. *Heart* **80**: 539–542.

45. Taylor CA, Fonte TA, Min JK. (2013) Computational fluid dynamics applied to cardiac computed tomography for noninvasive quantification of fractional flow reserve: scientific basis. *J Am Coll Cardiol* **61**: 2233–2241.

46. Benton SM, Tesche C, De Cecco CN *et al.* (2017) Noninvasive derivation of fractional flow reserve from coronary computed tomographic angiography: a review. *J Thorac Imaging* Aug 16. doi: 10.1097/RTI.0000000000000289.

47. Koo BK, Erglis A, Doh JH *et al.* (2011) Diagnosis of ischemia-causing coronary stenoses by noninvasive fractional flow reserve computed from coronary computed tomographic angiograms. Results from the prospective multicenter DISCOVER-FLOW (Diagnosis of ischemia-Causing Stenoses Obtained Via Noninvasive Fractional Flow Reserve) study. *J Am Coll Cardiol* **58**: 1989–1997.

48. Nakazato R, Park HB, Berman DS *et al.* (2013) Noninvasive fractional flow reserve derived from computed tomography angiography for coronary lesions of intermediate stenosis severity: results from the DeFACTO study. *Circ Cardiovasc Imaging* **6**: 881–889.

49. Nørgaard BL, Leipsic J, Gaur S *et al.* (2014) Diagnostic performance of noninvasive fractional flow reserve derived from coronary computed tomography angiography in suspected coronary artery disease: the NXT Trial (Analysis of Coronary Blood Flow Using CT Angiography: Next Steps). *J Am Coll Cardiol* **63**: 1145–1155.

50. Chung JH, Lee KE, Nam CW *et al.* (2017) Diagnostic performance of a novel method for fractional flow reserve computed from noninvasive computed tomography angiography (NOVEL-FLOW Study). *Am J Cardiol* **120**: 362–368.

51. Ko BS, Wong DTL, Norgaard BL *et al.* (2016) Diagnostic performance of transluminal attenuation gradient and noninvasive fractional flow reserve derived from 320-detector row CT angiography to diagnose hemodynamically significant coronary stenosis: An NXT substudy. *Radiology* **279**: 75–83.

52. Curzen NP, Nolan J, Zaman AG, Norgaard BL, Rajani R. (2016) Does the routine availability of CT-derived FFR influence management of patients with stable chest pain compared to CT angiography alone? The FFR$_{CT}$ RIPORD Study. *JACC Cardiovascular Imaging* **9**: 1188–1194.

53. Kim HJ, Vignon-Clementel IE, Coogan JS, Figueroa CA, Jansen KE, Taylor CA. (2010) Patient-specific modeling of blood flow and pressure in human coronary arteries. *Ann Biomed Eng* **38**: 3195–3209.

54. Lee KE, Kwon SS, Ji YC *et al.* (2016) Estimation of the flow resistances exerted in coronary arteries using a vessel length-based method. *Pflugers Arch-Eur J Physiol* **468**: 1449–1458.

55. Kwon SS, Chung EC, Park JS *et al.* (2014) A novel patient-specific model to compute coronary fractional flow reserve. *Prog Biophys Mol Biol* **116**: 48–55.

56. Wilson RF, Wyche K, Christensen BV, Zimmer S, Laxson DD. (1990) Effects of adenosine on human coronary arterial circulation. *Circulation* **82**: 1595–1606.

57. Coenen A, Lubbers MM, Kurate A *et al.* (2015) Fractional flow reserve computed from noninvasive CT angiography data: diagnostic performance of an on-site clinician-operated computational fluid dynamics algorithms. *Radiology* **274**: 674–683.

58. De Geer J, Sandstedt M, Bjorkholm A *et al.* (2016) Software-based on-site estimation of fractional flow reserve using standard coronary CT angiography data. *Acta Radiologica* **57**: 1186–1192.

59. Kawaji T, Shiomi H, Morishita H *et al.* (2017) Feasibility and diagnostic performance of fractional flow reserve measurement derived from coronary computed tomography angiography in real clinical practice. *Int J Cardiovasc Imaging* **33**: 271–281.

60. Ko BS, Cameron JD, Munnar RK *et al.* (2017) Noninvasive CT-derived FFR based on structural and fluid analysis: a comparison with invasive FFR for detection of functionally significant stenosis. *JACC Cardiovasc Imaging* **10**: 663–673.

61. Kruk M, Wardziak L, Demkow M *et al.* (2016) Workstation-based calculation of CTA-based FFR for intermediate stenosis. *JACC Cardiovasc Imaging* **9**: 690–699.

62. Renker M, Schoepf UJ, Wang R *et al.* (2014) Comparison of diagnostic value of a novel noninvasive coronary computed tomography angiography method versus standard coronary angiography for assessing fractional flow reserve. *Am J Cardiol* **114**: 1303–1308.

63. Tesche C, De Cecco CN, Caruso D *et al.* (2016) Coronary CT angiography derived morphological and functional quantitative plaque markers correlated with invasive fractional flow reserve for detecting hemodynamically significant stenosis. *J Cardiovasc Comput Tomogr* **10**: 199–206.

64. Wang R, Renker M, Schoepf UJ *et al.* (2016) Diagnostic value of quantitative stenosis predictors with coronary CT angiography compared to invasive fractional flow reserve. *Eur J Radiol* **84**: 1509–1515.

65. Yang DH, Kim YH, Roh JH *et al.* (2017) Diagnostic performance of on-site CT-derived fractional flow reserve versus CT perfusion. *Eur Heart J Cardiovasc Imaging* **18**: 432–440.

66. Baumann S, Renker M, Hetjens S *et al.* (2016) Comparison of coronary computed tomography-derived vs. invasive fractional flow reserve assessment: meta-analysis with subgroup evaluation of intermediate stenosis. *Acad Radiol* **23**: 1402–1411.

67. Danad I, Szymonifka J, Twisk JWR *et al.* (2017) Diagnostic performance of cardiac imaging methods to diagnose ischaemia-causing coronary artery disease when directly compared with fractional flow reserve as a reference standard: a meta-analysis. *Eur Heart J* **38**: 991–998.

68. Ding A, Qiu G, Lin W *et al.* (2016) Diagnostic performance of noninvasive fractional flow reserve derived from coronary computed tomography angiography in ischemia-causing coronary stenosis: a meta-analysis. *Jpn J Radiol* **34**: 795–808.

69. Gonzalez JA, Lipinkski MI, Flors L *et al.* (2015) Meta-analysis of diagnostic performance of coronary computed tomography angiography, computed tomography perfusion, and computed tomography-fractional flow reserve in functional myocardial ischemia assessment versus invasive fractional flow reserve. *Am J Cardiol* **116**: 1469–1478.

70. Li S, Peng L, Luo Y, Rong R, Liu J. (2015) The diagnostic performance of CT-derived fractional flow reserve for evaluation of myocardial ischaemia confirmed by invasive fractional flow reserve: a meta-analysis. *Clin Radiol* **70**: 476–486.

71. Wu W, Pan DR, Foin N *et al.* (2016) Noninvasive fractional flow reserve derived from coronary computed tomography angiography for identification of ischemic lesions: a systematic review and meta-analysis. *Sci Rep* **6**: 29409.

72. Xu R, Li C, Qian J, Ge J. (2015) Computed tomography-derived fractional flow reserve in the detection of lesion-specific ischemia. *Medicine* **94**: e1963.

73. Chu M, Dai N, Yang J, Westra J, Tu S. (2017) A systematic review of imaging anatomy in predicting functional significance of coronary stenoses determined by fractional flow reserve. *Int J Cardiovasc Imaging* **33**: 975–990.

74. Hwang D, Lee JM, Koo BK. (2016) Physiologic assessment of coronary artery disease: focus on fractional flow reserve. *Korean J Radiol* **17**: 307–320.

75. de Harder AM, Willemink MJ, De Jong *et al.* (2016) New horizons in cardiac CT. *Clin Radiol* **71**: 758–767.

76. Duguay TM, Tesche C, Vligenthart R *et al.* (2017) Coronary computed tomographic angiography-derived fractional flow reserve based on machine learning for risk stratification of non-culprit coronary narrowings in patients with acute coronary syndrome. *Am J Cardiol* **120**: 1260–1266.

77. Ri K, Kumamaru KK, Fujimoto S *et al.* (2017) Noninvasive computed tomography-derived fractional flow reserve based on structural and fluid analysis: reproducibility of on-site determination by unexpected observers. *J Comput Assist Tomogr* Sep 20. doi: 10.1097/RCT.0000000000000679.

78. Douglas PS, Pontone G, Hlatky MA *et al.* (2015) Clinical outcomes of fractional flow reserve by computed tomographic angiography-guided diagnostic strategies vs. usual care in patients with suspected coronary artery disease: the prospective longitudinal trial of FFRCT: outcome and resource impacts study. *Eur Heart J* **36**: 3359–3367.

79. Sun Z. (2015) The PLATFORM trial: an insight into the improved value of using FFRCT for reduction of invasive angiographic procedures. *Heart Res Open J* **2**: e13–e17.

80. Bilbey N, Blanke P, Naoum C *et al.* (2016) Potential impact of clinical use of noninvasive FFRCT on radiation dose exposure and downstream clinical event rate. *Clin Imaging* **40**: 1055–1060.

81. Assessing diagnostic value of non-invasive FFRCT in coronary care (ADVANCE) [Internet]. ClinicalTrials.Gov. Available from: https://clinicaltrials.gov/ct2/show/NCT02499679.

7 Summary and Conclusions

Coronary computed tomography angiography (CCTA) is a widely acceptable diagnostic imaging modality showing high diagnostic value in the diagnosis of coronary artery disease (CAD). The widespread use of CCTA as a less-invasive imaging modality in clinical practice is due to the rapid technological improvements in CT scanning techniques, which enable acquisition of high-resolution CCTA imaging datasets with minimal artifacts and, most important, low radiation dose. Currently, the radiation dose associated with CCTA is equivalent to or even lower than that of invasive coronary angiography (ICA). With the use of some recent dose-reduction strategies, radiation dose of CCTA is similar to that of chest X-ray examinations, thus making the CCTA a more attractive imaging modality.

The diagnostic value of CCTA not only lies in its ability to visualize and detect coronary arteries with excellent anatomical structures, but also to provide information beyond coronary lumen assessment. CCTA is able to characterize coronary plaques in terms of plaque composition, allowing for quantitative analysis of plaque features. This indicates that CCTA is superior to ICA, which is the gold standard for coronary lumen assessment. ICA is an excellent imaging technique for detecting arterial wall/lumen changes; however, its diagnostic value in assessing plaque components is limited. Analysis of plaque features is of clinical significance due to the association between plaque features and occurrence of major adverse cardiac events. In particular, some plaque characteristics such as low-attenuation plaque, non-calcified plaque, presence of spotty calcification, or other coronary lumen changes such as positive remodeling index

145

are identified on CCTA as indicators of high-risk plaques with clinical evidence showing the relationship between these plaque features and risk of developing major cardiac events. There is sufficient evidence showing that CCTA is comparable to intravascular ultrasound in the quantitative assessment of coronary plaques. Therefore, CCTA not only provides diagnostic value for CAD, but also offers information about the coronary plaque components that plays an important role in predicting major cardiac events through identifying the high-risk patients.

Despite significant improvements in both spatial and temporal resolution, most of the current CCTA applications lie in the demonstration of anatomical changes to the coronary artery lumen, while information about functional alterations to the coronary artery is limited due to the focus of this technique on lumen assessment. However, current research developments in the utilization of CCTA have enhanced the clinical value of this imaging technique, with the trend moving from the previously anatomy-focused approach to a combination of both anatomy and physiology assessments of CAD. This has led to increasing reports in CCTA-derived flow dynamic analysis.

CCTA-generated computational fluid dynamics (CFD) provides additional information about hemodynamic changes to the coronary artery tree when compared to the conventional approach of lumen assessment. Patient-specific CFD analysis is feasible with acquisition of high-resolution CCTA datasets and generation of realistic coronary geometry models with high precision. CFD simulations of coronary blood flow have shown the potential of detecting hemodynamics due to different types of plaques, with clinical significance of identifying high-risk or vulnerable plaques, thus augmenting diagnostic value of CCTA for determining significance of coronary lesions. Further, patient-specific CFD simulations demonstrate the improved diagnostic performance of CCTA with use of left coronary bifurcation angle when compared to CCTA lumen diagnosis, especially in the assessment of calcified coronary plaques. Incorporation of the measurement of the left coronary bifurcation angle into routine diagnostic approach is highly suggested to improve the diagnostic specificity and positive predictive value of CCTA.

The latest research direction of CCTA is to determine functional significance of coronary stenosis because coronary lumen stenosis or narrowing is a poor indicator for hemodynamic significance or myocardial ischemia. Thus, the paradigm shift of current CCTA applications lies in providing both anatomic and functional assessments of coronary lesions with the aim of detecting lesion-specific ischemia, therefore guiding effective patient management through identifying high-risk coronary lesions. This has led to the increasing application of CCTA-derived fractional flow reserve (FFR_{CT}). FFR_{CT} has represented another revolution of CT imaging in the diagnosis of CAD with promising results reported in the literature, based on multicenter and single-center studies. The most importance application of FFR_{CT} lies in the significant improvements in diagnostic performance of CCTA, mainly the higher specificity and positive predictive value than conventional CCTA. This is of paramount importance from a clinical perspective because the strategy of using FFR_{CT}-guided patient management results in reduction of unnecessary invasive procedures, while improving clinical outcomes and patient care.

This book has covered the aforementioned areas in detail, in particular the focus is given to the current research developments in CCTA-derived CFD and FFR_{CT} applications in the diagnostic assessment of significant CAD. Discussion on these areas are well supported by latest literatures, consisting of single-center, multicenter studies as well as systematic reviews and meta-analyses. Thus, it provides a useful and reliable resource for researchers who are interested in cardiac imaging, especially for those showing strong interests in coronary CT angiography. Challenges and limitations are also highlighted in these areas, which assist readers and researchers to conduct further research in this field.

Index